Michael Bonds, PhD

Race, Politics, and Community Development Funding
The Discolor of Mon~

"This book addresses one of the most critical political issues of the day—the impact of black elected officials on the allocation of public-services funds to black communities. The author reveals that simply electing a greater number of black officials does not automatically translate into gains for black communities, and that there may be some negative consequences of such electoral success.

Methodologically, this study illustrates the importance of qualitative research to flesh out the lessons learned (and occasionally hidden) by quantitative research. Although this book focuses on Milwaukee, the implication reaches well beyond any one community."

Gregory D. Squires
Professor of Sociology, Public Policy, and Public Administration,
George Washington University

"This study raises serious questions about the administration of federal funds for community development in inner-city Milwaukee, and confirms that favoritism of white CBOs existed at the expense of blacks CBOs in the years between 1975 and 1997, even where the latter were better managed. This book confirms the tendencies of cash-strapped mayors in this period to utilize CDBG funds for purposes other than for which the funding was meant. Top officials in Milwaukee permitted the diversion of funds from the poverty-stricken African-American community to other communities, marking an irony in a time of growth in the number of black elected officials.

Bonds explains that among the causative factors for resources being used in ways different than originally intended were not only racism, but a policy administration that was conducted in a bureaucracy lacking the needed number of black administrators with the capacity to intervene in such practices, allowing white officials to continue to distribute funds to non-black communities."

Ronald Walters, PhD
Professor, Government and Politics,
University of Maryland, College Park

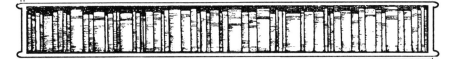

More pre-publication
REVIEWS, COMMENTARIES, EVALUATIONS . . .

"Michael Bonds' informative and provocative book tells of yet another American city governed by those who divide and conquer instead of unite and prosper. As cities all across the United States struggle with disinvestment and declining economies, Bonds takes the reader into a Milwaukee that uses its community development programs to further policies that exacerbate ethnic and racial tension, neighborhood competition, and the continued flight of capital.

In clear and concise prose, Bonds offers a thoroughly researched and expertly documented analysis of how the community development funding process can be hijacked by those who seek to protect their authority and bureaucratic turf at the expense of city residents. In the case of Milwaukee, and many other cities struggling with various forms of desegregation, the community development funding process pays lip service to the politics of inclusion, but operates as a vehicle for exclusion."

Rick Hornung
Learning Center Specialist,
Eastern Connecticut State University;
Author of *One Nation Under the Gun: Inside the Mohawk Civil War, At the Edge of All Things: In Search of Labrador,* and *Al Capone*

The Haworth Social Work Practice Press
An Imprint of The Haworth Press, Inc.
New York • London • Oxford

Race, Politics, and Community Development Funding
The Discolor of Money

HAWORTH Health and Social Policy
Marvin D. Feit, PhD

Maltreatment and the School-Age Child: Developmental Outcomes and Systems Issues by Phyllis T. Howing, John S. Wodarski, P. David Kurtz, and James Martin Gaudin Jr.

Health and Social Policy by Marvin D. Feit and Stanley F. Battle

Adolescent Substance Abuse: An Empirical-Based Group Preventive Health Paradigm by John S. Wodarski and Marvin D. Feit

Long-Term Care: Federal, State, and Private Options for the Future by Raymond O'Brien and Michael Flannery

Health and Poverty by Michael J. Holosko and Marvin D. Feit

Financial Management in Human Services by Marvin Feit and Peter Li

Race, Politics, and Community Development Funding: The Discolor of Money by Michael Bonds

Race, Politics, and Community Development Funding
The Discolor of Money

Michael Bonds, PhD

The Haworth Social Work Practice Press
An Imprint of The Haworth Press, Inc.
New York • London • Oxford

Published by

The Haworth Social Work Practice Press, an imprint of The Haworth Press, Inc., 10 Alice Street, Binghamton, NY 13904-1580.

PUBLISHER'S NOTE
Unless otherwise specified, quoted material ed from confidential
sources w͏ the research study.

Cover de͏

Library of Congress Cataloging-in-Publication Data

Bonds, Michael.
    Race, politics, and community development funding : the discolor of money / Michael Bonds.
      p. cm.
    Includes bibliographical references and index.
    ISBN 0-7890-2148-X (cloth : alk. paper)—ISBN 0-7890-2149-8 (pbk. : alk. paper)
    1. Community development—Wisconsin—Milwaukee. 2. Community Development Block Grant Program (U.S.) 3. African Americans—Wisconsin—Milwaukee—Politics and government. 4. Local government—Wisconsin. 5. African Americans—Wisconsin—Milwaukee—Social conditions. I. Title.
    HN80.M58B66 2004
    307.1'4'09775'95—dc21
                                       2003006745

CONTENTS

Foreword   vii

James Jennings

Acknowledgments   ix

Abbreviations   xi

Chapter 1. Introduction   1

Chapter 2. CDBG Program Overview   13

Chapter 3. The Socioeconomic Status of Milwaukee's African Americans   29

Chapter 4. Surveying the Impact of Race in Milwaukee's Allocation of CDBG Funds   39

Chapter 5. CDBG Allocation Patterns   55

Chapter 6. The Unequal and Ugly Effect of Race in the Allocation of CDBG Funds   75

Chapter 7. Bending Existing CDBG Rules   91

Chapter 8. Conclusion: How Race Directly Affects the Allocation of CDBG Funds in Milwaukee   101

Appendix A. Research Methods   113

References   117

Index   127

ABOUT THE AUTHOR

Michael Bonds, PhD, MPA, MS, is Assistant Professor in the Department of Educational Policy and Community Studies at the University of Wisconsin–Milwaukee (UWM). He teaches courses in Community Development, Community Problems, and Social Change. Dr. Bonds also worked as a Fiscal Analyst for the City of Milwaukee Common Council for eleven years and was the lead analyst to the Community Development Committee, Public Works Committee, Public Safety Committee, and Economic Development Committee. During these eleven years, he worked as the Community Development Block Grants Fiscal Analyst for eighteen months and reviewed proposals and recommendations for funding to the common council. He is recognized as an expert on the CDBG program, the topic of this book. Dr. Bonds co-authored a book titled *The State of Black Businesses in Milwaukee* (2000), and has written extensively on welfare reform in Wisconsin. Dr. Bonds served three years as a Scholar Practitioner with the Kellogg Foundation studying welfare reform in Wisconsin.

Foreword

This book represents one of the most serious and systematic efforts in the literature examining race and local politics and the distribution of municipal services. In addition, Michael Bonds revisits the question about the role and impact of black elected officials in cities with entrenched public service bureaucracies. In other words, do black elected officials make a difference in terms of the distribution of benefits? What, actually, is the impact of black political power on bureaucratic decisions regarding public benefits such as community development block grant funding for local organizations? Related to this, what is the role or impact of coalitions between blacks and liberal whites who gain electoral office in the distribution of municipal benefits?

This study is well researched in terms of the theoretical and historical literature and its focus on the city of Milwaukee. Dr. Bonds uses a sound theoretical framework to investigate the distribution of community development block grant funding in the city of Milwaukee. The author examines the distribution of $247 million between 1975 and 1997 as a case study for examining broader racial and class dynamics in this city. He utilizes data that reflect how the decisions and actions of government implicitly treat neighborhoods by race. The database includes surveys completed by community-based organizations, interviews with elected officials and government representatives, and analyses of program records. The author provides an insider's view of how decisions regarding neighborhoods are made in city hall. He spent considerable time in 1996 and 1997 working with city government and assisted with the evaluation of CDBG proposals and funding recommendations.

One conclusion of this study reminds us that the election of African Americans, and even the adoption of public policy aimed at assisting the economic and community development of neighborhoods, does not necessarily guarantee a favorable distribution of policy-related benefits. The author reminds us that the rhetoric and intent of public policy may not necessarily lead to a prescribed way of doing business regarding a particular policy. The implementation of public policy may look very different, indeed even inconsistent, with the intent of policy.

Although several contextual and political factors were favorable to African-American interests in Milwaukee, the actual distribution of CDBG dollars was skewed toward community-based organizations not controlled by, or serving, this group. This is related to a second and very important implication of Dr. Bonds' study: the arena for black political empowerment should not be confined simply to electoral politics. At the local level, the status and well-being of community-based organizations serving African Americans is critical in terms of guaranteeing racial and ethnic equality in the distribution of public goods. How certain kinds of mediating institutions involved with human services, education, job training, youth, and other services fare in the overall political and bureaucratic processes of a city is as important, if not more in some cases, than who gets elected to office.

This work is a model for others interested in examining the distribution of municipal services in places that have history of racial and ethnic conflict. Dr. Bonds' work is an important contribution to an earlier literature that focused on how race, class, and political variables influenced government decision making in the distribution of local goods. The study represents an effective model for examining the role of race and politics in the everyday decision making of urban bureaucracies.

James Jennings
Professor of Urban and Environmental
Policy and Planning
Tufts University

Acknowledgments

My accomplishment of this completed book, *Race, Politics, and Community Development Funding: The Discolor of Money,* is due in part to the input and reactions of many individuals. First, I thank the staff at the City of Milwaukee Community Block Grant Administration (CBGA) for providing me with unlimited access to their community development block grant (CDBG) records. Second, I am especially grateful to the staff of The Haworth Press who assisted in making this book a reality. Third, I am indebted to friends, colleagues, and scholars who read portions of this book and provided meaningful input. Finally, special thanks go to K.I.M. for their continued support during this project.

ABBREVIATIONS

AFDC	Aid for Families with Dependent Children
CAC	Citizen Advisory Committee
CBD	Central Business District
CBGA	Community Block Grant Administration
CBO	Community-Based Organization
CDA	Community Development Administration
CDBG	Community Development Block Grant
CDPC	Community Development Policy Committee
CHPC	Community Housing and Preservation Corporation
CIP	Capital Improvement Projects
COWSA	Community Organizing Westside Agency
CR-SDC	Community Relations-Social Development Commission
DCD	Department of City Development
EEOC	U.S. Equal Employment Opportunity Commission
ESHAC	East Side Housing Action Committee
F&P	Finance and Personnel Committee
FAP	Funding Allocation Plan
GA	Milwaukee County's General Assistance Program
HOME	Home Ownership Made Easy
HPC	Housing Partnership Corporation
HUD	Housing and Urban Development
ICRC	Inner City Redevelopment Corporation
MCC	Milwaukee Christian Center
MHAC	Milwaukee Housing Assistance Corporation
MUFBH	Milwaukee United for Better Housing
MUL	Milwaukee Urban League
NAC	Neighborhood Advisory Council
NIP	Neighborhood Improvement Project
NWSCDC	Northwest Side Community Development Corporation
RACM	Redevelopment Authority of the City of Milwaukee
RFP	Request for Proposal
SCO	South Community Organization
SDC	Social Development Commission
SMSA	Standard Metropolitan Statistical Area
TIN	Targeted Investment Neighborhood
WCC	Westside Conservation Corporation
ZN&D	Zoning, Neighborhoods, and Development Committee

Chapter 1

Introduction

Since W. E. B. DuBois wrote about "the color line" serving as the defining issue of the twentieth century, social scientists have created a vast literature revolving around the study of race, and its impact on the politics of "who gets what and how." Throughout the first sixty years of the twentieth century, scholars followed Dr. DuBois' lead to chronicle how a system of legalized segregation skewed the distribution and allocation of wealth and resources. Following decades of struggle that included protest, litigation, and legislation, the Jim Crow system began to crumble and social scientists seized the opportunity to investigate how the emerging African-American political power could affect the delivery of municipal services and the distribution of municipal resources to constituents who were once openly locked out and turned aside at city hall.

That is the focus of this research—to investigate how the politics of race in Milwaukee, Wisconsin, determined the distribution of more than $247 million of community development block grant (CDBG) funds during the period 1975 to 1997 (see Table 1.1). A federal program enacted by Congress in August 1974, the CDBG process awards funds to local communities based on a multiple-need formula that considers housing, population, and poverty measures. Passed by Congress during the height of the Watergate scandal and the American withdrawal from the war in Vietnam, the CDBG program was intended to reform and consolidate seven programs initiated as part of the "Great Society" legislation of the 1960s: Urban Renewal, Model Cities, Water and Sewer Facilities Grants, Neighborhood Facilities Grants, Public Facilities Loans, Open Space Land Grants, and Rehabilitation Loans (Nathan et al., 1977; United States Department of Housing and Urban Development [HUD], 1996). This change provided local governments with more flexibility in using federal trans-

TABLE 1.1. Distribution of Community Development Block Grants in Milwaukee from 1975 to 1997

Year	CDBG (per $1,000)
1975-1976	13,383
1980-1981	22,794
1985-1986*	17,684
1988	25,090
1989	15,362
1990	15,328
1991	14,342
1992	16,233
1993	16,101
1994	20,500
1995	22,000
1996	24,274
1997	24,705
Total	247,796

Source: CBGA (various years)

*Switched from a fiscal year to calendar year

fer payments for program activities such as housing, employment, recreation, and social services aimed at eliminating poverty and blight.

To fully examine how racial considerations influenced one local government's decisions regarding the allocation and distribution of these funds, this research focuses on five basic research questions:

1. Does race play a role in the distribution of CDBG funds in Milwaukee?
2. Does the presence of African-American elected officials on the Community Development Policy Committee (CDPC), the policy-making body for the CDBG program, affect the distribution of CDBG funds to majority African-American neighborhoods and African-American community-based organizations (CBOs)?
3. Does an increased number of African-American elected officials result in more CDBG funds being allocated to African-American communities and African-American CBOs?

4. Does the election of a Caucasian liberal mayor and liberal Caucasian council members who express concern for or interest in the plight of African-American neighborhoods affect the distribution of CDBG funds to those areas?
5. What are the implications of these CDBG allocation decisions for African-American neighborhoods and African-American CBOs?

Hopefully, the answers to these questions will provide a greater understanding both of the CDBG process in Milwaukee, and more generally, of the ways in which race colors how millions of CDBG dollars are distributed each year.

By employing a variety of methods, including open rebellion against federal, state, and local governments, mass movement peaceful protests, voter registration drives, and litigation and legislation, African Americans have dramatically increased their ability to represent themselves as city councilors, mayors, and members of congress. Throughout the last half of the twentieth century, political participation has been viewed as an important vehicle for enacting favorable government policies that improve the quality of life in African-American communities.

This increased presence of African Americans in the political machinery of federal, state, and local governments led to a number of favorable rulings from the United States Supreme Court designed to weaken the old Jim Crow barriers and enforce constitutional protections regarding voting and due process. Though plaintiffs brought these cases out of protest battles and years of petitioning elected officials for redress, the nonelected, federal judiciary has been one of the most significant catalysts toward effecting the changes that created conditions for greater African-American participation in the political process. In *Guinn v. United States* (1915), the United States Supreme Court ruled that the grandfather clause was unconstitutional, and it was therefore prohibited (Jaynes and Williams, 1989; Perry and Parent, 1995). This was the first step toward abolishing state-mandated sanctions that barred African-American voters from the polls. Similarly, the United States Supreme Court ruled in *Smith v. Allwright* (1944) that an all-white primary was unconstitutional (Bell, 1980). In the *Brown v. Board of Education* ruling of 1954, the Court outlawed school segregation and provided African Americans with another vehicle for advancing their participation in the political arena (Perry and Parent, 1995). In the 1966 case, *South Carolina v. Katzenbach,* the justices upheld the Voting Rights Act of 1965 as a legitimate exercise of Congress's power to rid the nation of racial discrimination (Combs, 1995). In 1968, these protections were further extended when the Court prohibited the states from changing certain types of voter qualification laws without the permission of a federal court or the United States Department of Justice (Davidson, 1984).

In response to these rulings and the continued stream of protest that stretched through the 1950s and 1960s, the executive and legislative branches of federal, state, and local governments enacted hundreds of new laws, regulations, and ordinances designed to improve African Americans' access to the mechanisms of government. Across the country, most state and local governments took the initiative after Congress passed laws that expressly targeted the discriminatory practices that dated back to the days of Jim Crow if not earlier.

In the aftermath of the use of federal troops to integrate schools in Little Rock, Arkansas, and in direct response to Governor Orville Faubus' defiance of the United States Supreme Court and President Dwight Eisenhower, Congress passed the Civil Rights Act of 1957 which allowed African Americans to file lawsuits challenging racial discrimination regarding the right to vote (Combs, 1995; Perry and Parent, 1995). The landmark Civil Rights Act of 1964 explicitly guaranteed African Americans access to all public accommodations and higher education, and offered antidiscrimination safeguards for privately employed workers. By directly addressing the issue of political participation by racial minorities, this law furthered African Americans' voting rights in the South by prohibiting the use of literacy tests or formal education to determine voting qualifications (Combs, 1995; Jaynes and Williams, 1989; Perry and Parent, 1995).

Despite the protections offered by these civil rights laws, Congress went a step further to directly intervene in the effort to register African-American voters. By passing the Voting Rights Act of 1965, lawmakers authorized federal marshals to summarily register African Americans in the states and counties in the South where less than 50 percent of the voting age population was registered to vote in the 1964 presidential election. Moreover, the 1965 Voting Rights Act authorized the United States attorney general to file suit in federal court challenging the enforcement of poll taxes in states and local elections in the South. For the first time in American history, the federal government was directed by Congress to use the federal courts to openly challenge states and municipalities that held on to discriminatory voter registration practices (Combs, 1995; Jaynes and Williams, 1989; Parker, 1990; Perry and Parent, 1995).

The United States Congress would later grant extensions to the Voting Rights Act of 1965 in 1970, 1975, and 1982. In 1982, the Voting Rights Act of 1965 was extended twenty-five years and provided a statistic showing that patterns of racial discrimination continued as many states and localities used voter dilution tactics to weaken the power of neighborhoods, towns, and counties that were predominantly African-American. The 1982 extension also helped increase the African-American presence in politics by allowing a plaintiff to seek a remedy for discrimination even if he or she could not prove a local or state government's "intent" to discriminate. This reform allowed African Americans to sue dozens of local and state governments on the grounds that their policies, practices, and laws had the inadvertent or unintended consequence of strengthening the power of Caucasian voters at the expense of African Americans (Derfner, 1984).

The aforementioned congressional and judicial efforts have resulted in an increased level of political involvement by African Americans. The number of African-American elected officials has increased significantly since 1965 when there were fewer than 500 African-American elected officials in the United States. In 1970, the number increased to 1,469, and it would further increase to 7,225 by 1989 (Hanks, 1987; Jaynes and Williams, 1989; Parker 1990; Pohlmann, 1990; Williams, 1990).

In addition to the number of African Americans elected to public offices, the number of African Americans registered to vote increased significantly. The number of African Americans registered to vote in southern states increased by more than 5.6 million voters, from 1,511,000 in 1940 to 5,842,000 in 1988. The biggest growth occurred during the decade 1965 to 1975, when more than four million southern African Americans registered (Jaynes and Williams, 1989; Perry and Parent, 1995). With this increased political power, African Americans expected an increase in federal government benefits, state-sponsored protections, and municipal services.

Despite this growth on the voting rolls, many scholars and researchers have conducted studies that dispute the effectiveness of whether increased participation in the accepted political machinery leads to a proportionate increase in the distribution of revenues and delivery of services. On the one hand, some studies indicate that increased African-American political power results in more benefits for African-American communities. These benefits include increased employment opportunities, increased municipal services (fire, police, garbage collection), increased share of municipal contracts, increased representation on citizen boards, and an increased number of commissions (Browning et al., 1984; Eisinger, 1982; Green and Wilson, 1989; Hanks, 1987; Headley, 1985; Jones, 1978; MacManus, 1990; Morris, 1984; Perry, 1980; Robinson, 1990).

Several studies have identified benefits obtained by African Americans in specific cities, when African Americans dominated the political structure. Beauregard (1990) noted that there was an increase in the percentage of African Americans employed by city government once African-American politicians were elected mayors in the cities he studied. Similarly, MacManus (1990) found that the percentage of municipal contracts awarded to African Americans increased in cities in which African-American mayors gained political control.

Other researchers have shown that increased African-American political power does not necessarily result in more benefits to African-American communities. Instead, they argued that African-American political power was limited by the following factors:

1. Local demographic and structural changes (loss of manufacturing jobs, a shift to a service economy, a rise in high-tech jobs, and white flight) had a devastating impact on African-American communities.
2. A declining tax base and the loss of federal funds at a time when African Americans gained political power in cities weakened black political power.
3. The public's negative attitude toward redistribution policies and the impact that such policies can have on the community's tax base also undermined black political power.
4. In the face of hostility from several established constituencies, African-American politicians overlooked their voter base and found themselves preoccupied with responding to the business

community's concerns (Beauregard, 1990; Bobo and Gilliam, 1990; Cross, 1987; Green and Wilson, 1989; Piliawsky, 1985; Piven and Clowards, 1971).

Of particular importance are several studies of the recent political structure in Atlanta, Georgia, where researchers found that African-American dominance of the political structure did not lead to a complete transfer into proportionate benefits for many in the African-American community. These studies noted that Mayor Maynard Jackson and Mayor Andrew Young were able to provide some contracts and employment opportunities to only the city's African-American middle class, bringing only marginal benefits to poor African-American residents (Jones, 1978; White, 1992).

Although there is vast, contemporary research literature on the effect of African-American political power, increased voter registration, and growing numbers of elected officials on the African-American community, there are few studies on the role of racial politics and its effects on the bureaucratic machinery of distributing municipal services in large cities. In short, there are a number of gaps in this research. Many studies focused on the role of the executive branch (mayor) of city government, neglecting the legislative branch's role in public policy decisions on the distribution of urban services. This research will avoid this limitation by including the legislative branch, common council, and examining its impact on the distribution of CDBG funds.

Most research on the role of racial politics in the distribution of urban services has focused on macrolevel issues (employment, housing, education, the economy), areas over which the private sector has much more influence and control than the public sector. This research will instead focus on a microlevel issue, the CDBG program, an area where the private sector has less influence in the distribution of CDBG funds.

Still, most prior studies of African-American political power have focused on the number of African Americans elected to office. All too often, these studies contend that a mere increase in the number of African-American city councilors, mayors, or members of Congress represents a net gain of power. But winning an election is only one result and one indicator of power. This research will look at another result and indicator—whether winning local elections for the city council and changes in the mayoralty lead to a significant increase in the amount of CDBG funds allocated to programs that target improvement of African-American neighborhoods or community-based organizations that are rooted in servicing the African-American community. In short, this study seeks to fill the research gaps by examining how African-American elected officials specifically influence the distribution of CDBG funds toward their African-American constituents.

Milwaukee is an interesting case to examine the impact of racial politics on the distribution of CDBG funds. Between 1975 and 1997, Milwaukee experienced major demographic and political changes, which had significant implications for the city's African Americans and the delivery of urban services. Though many other cities experienced similar changes, Milwaukee's particular politics and geography allow for a researcher to track the possible correlation between race and the allocation of CDBG funds.

The city's African-American population grew dramatically during the study period. In 1975, African Americans comprised 18 percent of the city's total population, but grew to 30.4 percent by 1990 (United States Department of Commerce, Bureau of Census). As a result of this population growth, there was an increase in African-American political power.

In addition to the growth in the number of African Americans in Milwaukee, the number of African-American council members in Milwaukee increased from two of sixteen (12.5 percent) in 1975 to five of seventeen (29.4 percent) by 1992. Thus, for the first time in the city's history, the percentage (29.4 percent) of African Americans serving on the city council nearly reflected their proportion of the city's total population, 30.4 percent (Proceedings of the Common Council, 1975 to 1976, 1988 to 1989, and 1991 to 1992).

The increased number of African Americans elected to the common council provided the African-American community with several advantages. In terms of absolute numbers and percentages, the African-American community was now strongly represented on the common council. African-American common council members now had more opportunities for representation on various council committees, such as the CDPC. The increased number of African-American common council members provided them with more political clout to obtain benefits for their aldermanic districts. The challenge was to

use this increased political power to provide districts with more benefits, such as a greater share of CDBG funds.

In 1988, Henry Maier, then the longest serving mayor of any major
U.S. city (1960 to 1988) retired, which provided an opportunity for
the city to elect its first new mayor since the federal and state government enacted many of the reforms created in the wake of the Civil
Rights Movement. For most African-American voters, Mayor Maier
was considered to be a hostile presence at city hall. He opposed an
open-housing ordinance; he refused to intervene in the school desegregation dispute of 1970 despite requests from African-American
leaders; and he opposed scattered low-income housing sites. Besides
these open policy disputes with African-American voters, Mayor
Maier further angered them by strongly supporting a Caucasian
police chief who was disliked by a large segment of the city's African-American community. Many African-American voters viewed
the mayor's repeated support for the chief as a direct reminder of his
aggressive response to the 1967 riot, which resulted in the calling out
of the National Guard and imposition of a curfew (Eisinger 1976;
Gruberg, 1990).

In addition to neglecting the concerns of African-American residents, Mayor Maier appointed few African Americans to decision-
making positions. During his twenty-eight years as mayor, he did not
appoint any African-American department heads and only one served
as an administrator (out of eighty-one local administrators). Furthermore, only twenty-eight (7.2 percent) of 387 people that Mayor
Maier appointed to various city boards and commissions were African Americans (Community Relations-Social Development Commission [CR-SDC] and Milwaukee Urban League [MUL], 1970).

With the election of a new mayor in 1988, the executive branch's
response to African Americans' concerns changed. Voters selected
State Senator John O. Norquist as mayor over former acting Governor Martin Schreiber. Norquist won all three majority African-American aldermanic districts, votes that his opponent had counted on
(Umhoefer, 1988; Walters, 1988). At the outset, Mayor Norquist rewarded the city's African-American community for its political support. He appointed an unprecedented number of African Americans
to cabinet-level positions and as top administrators in his first administration.

Mayor Norquist's ability to "reward" the African-American community through the appointment process was facilitated by a change in state law. In 1988, the Wisconsin State Legislature modified a state law to allow the mayor more appointment power in city government. Mayor Norquist appointed African-American heads of departments such as City Development; Employee Relations; Fire and Police Commission; Public Works; Purchasing; and other high-level administrative positions (Mitchell, 1994). Another change was that African Americans increased their share of the city's workforce from 16.1 percent in 1980 to 20.3 percent in 1990, an increase that occurred despite a reduction in the municipal workforce of 400 employees from 1986 to 1990 (Eisinger, 1991).

Along with a change in the mayor and an increase in the number of African-American council members, the legislative body underwent changes that saw the election of some Caucasian members who were more sympathetic to the needs of the African-American community than some of their predecessors. Caucasian community activists Tom Donegan, Mary Anne McNulty, and Paul Henningsen were elected to the council in 1983 to 1984 and Lorraine McNamara-McGraw was elected in 1989. These individuals were generally supportive of policies designed to improve conditions in the city's African-American community (Gruberg, 1990; Proceedings of the Common Council, 1989).

Some might argue that these changes would lead to African Americans receiving an increased share of CDBG funds to improve conditions in the African-American community. For the reasons previously noted, it appeared reasonable to expect that between 1975 and 1997 CDBG dollars flowing into Milwaukee's African-American CBOs and African-American neighborhoods would increase. During this period, the African-American population increased markedly, both in absolute and relative terms—and a host of social and economic indicators convincingly demonstrated the critical need to address various social and economic ills. Also, in the first half of the period (1975-1988), Mayor Henry Maier—whose relationship with the African-American community was strained at best and hostile at worst over his twenty-eight-year term—governed Milwaukee. In contrast, in 1988, John O. Norquist was elected mayor with a great deal of support from the African-American community. His initial appointments of African Americans and his public policies gave every indication of sensitivity to the plight of the city's African Americans. In addition, turnover in the city council appeared to be more favorable to African Americans. Not only did the number of African-American council members increase from two of sixteen to five of seventeen, but also a number of Caucasian progressives, some with long ties to the African-American community, were elected. Given these trends, it seemed plausible to expect that more CDBG dollars would be awarded to African-American neighborhoods and African-American CBOs.

Chapter 1 of this book reviews African Americans' struggle to obtain political power by examining the role that the U.S. Supreme Court, U.S. Congress, and black boycott methods, such as picketing, marches, and sit-ins, played in providing African Americans with increased power and the impact of these efforts.

Chapter 2 contains an overview of the CDBG program—its origins, history, and development, and provides a presentation of the reasons why the CDBG program was chosen for study. This chapter summarizes prior research on how Milwaukee and other communities allocated their CDBG monies and who appears to have the most influence in these decisions.

Chapter 3 outlines the socioeconomic conditions confronting Milwaukee's African Americans. Census data coupled with a substantial amount of research highlight the extreme degree of segregation, relative poverty, unemployment, and exclusion from political and economic power of African Americans in Milwaukee. In portraying the state of African Americans in Milwaukee, this chapter has three objectives: First, it will provide a general description of Milwaukee's African-American population from 1975 to 1995. Second, it will review major socioeconomic indicators, which clearly show that a sizeable share of Milwaukee's African-American population lives in very distressed and impoverished neighborhoods. Third, the chapter will discuss how the city's African-American community can benefit from the CDBG program.

Chapter 4 discusses results of mail surveys to CBOs, and interviews with elected officials and representatives of CBOs and public bureaucracies conducted to obtain their views on the role that race played in the distribution of CDBG funds in Milwaukee between 1975 to 1997.

Chapter 5 provides a quantitative test of the prominent figures in the CDBG funding process and offers findings from the "trace analysis" of the CDBG proposals. The goal was to determine which steps in the CDBG process are most critical. Who is the most prominent figure? Is it the mayor, as most respondents seem to think? Has this changed over time? In addition to reporting the results of this survey, the chapter examines and analyzes how applications for CDBG funds are handled from the proposal stage to the final allocation decisions. This analysis intends to identify who wields the power to allocate funds. As a corollary to this analysis, this chapter investigates the CDBG distribution patterns by aldermanic districts. Geographically based criteria are needed to help the study establish the degree to which the African-American community gained from the CDBG program. The chapter concludes with a comparison of allocation patterns under the administration of two very different mayors.

Chapter 6 draws upon interviews, analyses of program records, and results from eighteen months (April 1996 to October 1997) as a participant observer in the CDBG allocation process.

Chapter 7 illustrates how existing rules were modified to benefit Caucasian CBOs while African-American CBOs were penalized. This included a review of carry-over requests, contract extension requests, reprogramming dollar requests, recommended funding for ineligible groups, and so forth.

Chapter 8 provides a summary of the research findings and their implications for Milwaukee's African-American community as well as African-American communities in other cities.

Chapter 2

CDBG Program Overview

The CDBG is a federally funded program enacted in August 1974 as Public Law 93-383. The CDBG program consolidated seven previously funded federal programs:

1. Urban Renewal
2. Model Cities
3. Water and Sewer Facilities Grants
4. Neighborhood Facilities Grants
5. Public Facilities Loans
6. Open Space Land Grants
7. Rehabilitation Loans (Nathan et al., 1977)

This change provided local governments with more flexibility in using federal transfer payments for program activities (housing, employment, recreation, social services, etc.). The CDBG Program awards funds to local communities based on a multiple-need formula that considers housing, population, and poverty measures.

The consolidation of these seven programs was viewed as a means to better allocate federal funds to local communities for several reasons. One advantage was that it provided local officials with more discretion on establishing the use of CDBG funds for program activities, and it allowed for social and geographical targeting within broad federal guidelines. Another advantage was that it streamlined the CDBG application process. It required only one CDBG application for all CDBG activities instead of an application for each proposed activity. Furthermore, it reduced the inflexibility and duplication of overlapping and administrative burdens that other federal programs presented. Finally, it provided certainty of funding by awarding

CDBG funds to government units on a formula basis rather than by an administrative decision (Dommel and Associates, 1982; Rich, 1993).

Besides these improvements, the CDBG program incorporated seven national objectives when it was created:

1. The elimination of slums and blight and the prevention of blighting influences and the deterioration of property and neighborhood and community facilities of importance to the welfare of the community, principally persons of low and moderate income;
2. The elimination of conditions, which are detrimental to health, safety, and public welfare, through code enforcement, demolition, interim rehabilitation assistance, and related activities;
3. The conservation and expansion of the Nation's housing stock in order to provide a decent home and a suitable living environment for all persons, but principally those of low and moderate income;
4. The expansion and improvement of the quantity and quality of community services, principally for persons of low and moderate income, which are essential for sound community development and for the development of viable urban communities;
5. A more rational utilization of land and other natural resources and the better arrangement of residential, commercial, industrial, recreational, and other needed activity centers;
6. The reduction of the isolation of income groups within communities and geographical areas and the promotion of an increase in the diversity and vitality of neighborhoods through the spatial deconcentration of housing opportunities for persons of lower income and the revitalization of deteriorating or deteriorated neighborhoods to attract persons of higher income; and
7. The restoration and preservation of properties of special value for historic, architectural, or esthetic reasons. (Nathan et al., 1977, p. 53)

Since its inception in 1974, the CDBG program has undergone numerous changes. Two philosophical approaches held by different presidential administrations toward the CDBG program, i.e., "hands-off" and "hands-on," characterized these changes. On the one hand, some presidents (Ford, Reagan, and Bush Sr.) took a "hands-off" approach to the distribution of CDBG funds. They left it up to local communities to decide how to use CDBG funds within broader federal guidelines. To allow for such discretion, CDBG decisions were left to the local government units. This resulted in the elimination of: some monitoring, oversight, and compliance requirements; programs and benefit requirements for low- and moderate-income communities; and the inception of vague legislative directives relative to cities' use of CDBG funds which allowed them to interpret the meaning of those directives. Such a "hands-off" approach resulted in less CDBG funds being directed toward low- and moderate-income communities and more going to regular citywide projects (Dommel, 1980; Dommel, 1984; Rich, 1993; Rosenfeld, 1980).

On the other side of the debate, some presidents (Carter, Clinton) took a more "hands-on" approach toward the CDBG program. They emphasized greater federal involvement in monitoring the use of CDBG funds and in targeting them to low- and moderate-income communities, and requiring public participation in local government units' CDBG decision-making processes (Dommel, 1980; Dommel, 1984; Rich, 1993; Rosenfeld, 1980; Vacha, personal communication, 1997).

For a number of interrelated reasons, the CDBG program offered an excellent opportunity to examine the distribution of discretionary funds by those "who govern" and to identify the implications of these decisions for African-American CBOs and African-American neighborhoods. For instance, the CDBG program provided local officials with considerable flexibility in deciding their CDBG program's activities (Orlebeke, 1983). The CDBG program also represented a new source of funding for some local government units that had not participated previously in categorical programs that could pay for the operating costs of social programs (youth, employment, home counseling). Prior to the CDBG program, many local government units had not budgeted, or had insufficiently budgeted, for such programs. Likewise, the CDBG program represented the largest federal revenue source most local government units received, and it did not require a local "match" or tax-levy funds as a condition for receiving this aid. In addition, the CDBG program was used as leverage for other funds for housing and economic-development-related activities. A further aspect of the CDBG program that made it an attractive source of revenue for local government was the Section 108 program. Cities used the Section 108 program to borrow as much as three times their future CDBG allotments for short-term economic and community development projects. Finally, another CDBG leveraging device was the "CD float" which allowed CDBG entitlement communities to draw down their unexpended funds from previous CDBG funds to create a capital pool for short-term, private sector economic development projects (Dommel, 1984; Liebschutz, 1983; Orlebeke, 1983).

Numerous individuals are involved in the distribution of CDBG funds. Among these are mayors, city councilors, civil servants, CBOs, and citizens. Their roles in the distribution of CDBG funds vary from one community to another. The distribution of urban services is strongly influenced by politicians in local communities. The mayor has been considered the dominant political figure in the CDBG funding process. Prior research indicated that mayors find methods to reward groups that supported them. Cingranelli (1981) contended that mayors were responsive to areas that provided them with potential support in their previous elections. Numerous studies have documented that mayors dominated the CDBG distribution in local communities. Mayors have used the following techniques to dominate the CDBG program:

1. hiring political allies and supporters as paid consultants;
2. rewarding supporters with recommendations for CDBG-funded projects, and not recommending funding for nonsupporters;
3. appointing supporters as representatives to key CDBG-funding committees;
4. co-opting dissenting groups opposed to the mayor on major projects by awarding them CDBG projects; and
5. using CDBG funds to pay for city projects and positions that were usually funded with tax-levy dollars (Blumenfield, 1988; Orlebeke, 1983; Schamndt et al., 1983; Wong and Peterson, 1986).

Mayors are able to exert this influence over the CDBG program for several reasons. In most cities, they have the power to appoint the CDBG director, the individual who oversees the day-to-day operations of the CDBG program. This person is accountable to the mayor.

Mayors can appoint citizens and representatives to important policy and citizen committees related to the CDBG program. On top of this direct power, mayors form coalitions with city councilors who push for their pet projects. Moreover, the federal government recognizes mayors as the key figures in city government for administering the CDBG program. Finally, most mayors have the ability to appoint people to high-paying jobs in order to compensate them for their political support (Dommel and Associates, 1982; Harrigan, 1989).

Research has shown that different mayors, just as different presidents, have used the CDBG program differently. In Chicago, the use of CDBG funds by types of activities and targeting efforts were found to have changed over four mayoral administrations (Richard Daley/ Michael Bilandic; Jane Byrne; Harold Washington; and Richard Daley Jr.). The relationship between total block grant spending and overall community need was strongest under the Daley's/Bilandic's administrations (r = .60) and weakest during Byrne's years (r = .38), with both the Washington (r = .54) and Daley Jr. (r = .51) administrations showing moderately strong relationships (Rich, 1993).

Some mayors put different emphasis on targeting CDBG funds to African-American neighborhoods than other mayors.

> Following the election of Harold Washington, the city's first African-American mayor, the geographic distribution of block grants funds was more responsive to community needs, and especially to the needs of African-American community areas, as seen in the moderately positive and statistically significant relationships between the percentage of blacks and CDBG expenditures during the Washington administration. (Rich, 1993, p. 208)

Other cities were found to be effective in targeting CDBG funds to African-American neighborhoods (Browning et al., 1984).

In Baltimore, Mayor William Donald Schaefer dominated the CDBG program by rewarding supporters of his development plans and co-opting opponents of it. The mayor punished groups that opposed his plans by withholding CDBG dollars from them (Peterson et al., 1986; Wong and Peterson, 1986). Other studies also found situations in which the mayor dominated the CDBG process (Orkelebe, 1983; Peterson et al., 1986; Rich, 1993; Wong and Peterson, 1986).

Prior research on the mayors' roles in the distribution of CDBG funds has several shortcomings. First, most of these studies focused on the outcome (actual dollars allocated) of CDBG decisions under different mayoral administrations rather than examining the CDBG decision-making process, and the role mayors played in that process. Dollars awarded are an important matter to study and this research will certainly analyze the pattern of funding in Milwaukee. Yet it is also important to understand the process involved in arriving at these outcomes. This research will examine each step of the CDBG decision-making process. A second shortcoming of previous research, with the exception of Chicago's studies, has been to focus on short time periods, one to four years, which may reflect atypical funding patterns, or patterns in which the same public officials made the funding decisions. This study will avoid this pitfall by studying a twenty-three-year period under two different mayors.

Along with mayors, city councilors play an important role in the distribution of CDBG funds. Common council members establish policies for CDBG activities; they serve on committees that review and approve CDBG funding and they designate the CDBG-eligibile geographic areas. Local lawmakers establish the city's CDBG application process for submittal of requests to HUD for CDBG funds and they influence citizen participation requirements. In many cities, the city councilors appoint citizens to various CDBG advisory committees, and advocate and vote for CDBG projects that help their aldermanic districts (Gleiber and Steger, 1983; Liebschutz, 1983; Schmandt et al., 1986; Steger, 1984).

Although common councils have a role in the CDBG allocation process in most cities, their roles have been minimal and passive when compared to other branches of government. In Chicago, prior to the election of Harold Washington as the city's first African-American mayor, the council exerted little influence or interest in the distribution of CDBG funds. Until Mayor Washington's term, aldermen avoided specific debates and intervention only to pass a routine ordinance approving the city's CDBG application (Rich, 1993). In St. Louis, common council members routinely passed only one resolution authorizing the submittal of the CDBG application to HUD (Schmandt et al., 1983).

Though these conclusions tend to illustrate the strength of the mayor via the council, the research is limited because researchers have not examined how local lawmakers chose to participate in the day-to-day funding decisions and administration of the CDBG program. This study will attempt to correct this shortcoming by studying actions of council members at the committee level and examining where funding decisions were broken down into specific line items and precise allocations for CBOs and other grant recipients.

Civil servants also influence the allocation of urban services. These men and women have several sources of power, which gives them influence in the distribution of urban services. One source of power is their use of nonlegislative, regulatory rules and procedures to either promote efficiency or determine service delivery. Jones (1981) suggested two rules: need and service conditions (characteristics of a community) to measure efficiency and effectiveness of their service delivery. He claimed that these nonelected, civil servants mixed and matched the principles of "rationality" and "satisficing" when deciding how to distribute services and allocate resources. The rational perspective indicated that policymakers adopt the most efficient method for a proportionate distribution of services. Satisficing indicates that policymakers are called upon to satisfy a variety of conflicting constituencies and create an acceptable distribution of services, which is not the most efficient.

In addition to these rules, civil servants made policy decisions on an incremental basis when policy decisions reflected marginal changes. Once established, existing practices were used to determine future decisions. The best indicator of a policy decision on expenditures in a community was the previous year's decisions (Cingranelli, 1981; Garvey, 1993).

Official discretion represented another method to determine service delivery patterns. Civil servants have used a range of decision-making powers to make public policies based on their expertise and technical capabilities, without external scrutiny. Civil servants have used their discretion to assist them in achieving these tasks (Bryner, 1987; Garvey, 1993).

The role of civil servants in deciding service allocation is directly related to the distribution of CDBG funds for several reasons. They administer the decision rules, procedures, and guidelines for distributing CDBG funds. Afterward, they are responsible for implementing, monitoring, and evaluating the performance of CBOs and city agencies that receive CDBG dollars. Moreover, civil servants provide technical assistance and advice to CBOs seeking CDBG dollars. Finally, public agencies make CDBG recommendations to elected officials (Ellison et al., 1986; Gleiber and Steger, 1983; Judd and Mush-katel, 1982; Steger, 1984).

The physical, economic, and social needs of a community have been used to determine if CDBG funds were being allocated to low- and moderate-income areas per HUD's requirements. Bunce and Goldberg (1979) created an index of community need using the seven national objectives of the CDBG program as the basis for selecting twenty need indicators (e.g., poverty, housing, unemployment, crime, and density) expressed in either percentage or per-capita terms. These twenty measures included direct indicators of community needs, so-cioeconomic variables associated with urban blight, substandard housing, and measures of economic and population loss.

Although a variety of indicators have been used to measure com-munity need, most need variables have been used as part of an index of community need. Bunce and Goldberg (1979) created a three-dimensional need index from the twenty community need variables previously mentioned, using indicators such as age and decline, den-sity, and poverty. Other researchers have used a need index to study the distribution of CDBG funds (Bunce and Goldberg, 1979; Bunce and Glickman, 1980; Dommel and Rich, 1987; Gleiber and Steger, 1983).

The use of need indicators has several shortcomings. Need indica-tors reflect only the measures of conditions in a community, but do not explain the decision-making process used to award funds to needy areas. Furthermore, need indicators may be too standardized to accurately reflect the need of the local environment where those funds were being distributed. This study seeks to avoid these prob-lems by identifying the needs of a local area and then examining the decision-making process to determine if the neediest areas, Milwau-kee's African-American neighborhoods, received their fair share of CDBG funds.

Community-based organizations play a crucial role in the distribu-tion of urban services. CBOs can stimulate service demands on gov-ernment units by requesting or demanding that specific services be provided for a particular neighborhood. CBOs may be able to take advantage of special rules, either explicit or implicit, that result in better services for some neighborhoods. If government units are more sensitive to demands from neighborhoods represented by strong CBOs, then the link between citizens and municipal output will be strengthened. Moreover, CBOs can facilitate government regulations by intervening in the compliance process (Jones, 1981).

CBOs play a number of specific roles in the CDBG allocation process itself. CBOs lobby elected officials and public officials to fund projects in their districts or projects that affect their districts. In addition, CBOs can help identify community need and assist in the technical preparation of CDBG applications. CBOs can further serve as liaisons between their neighborhoods and the public bureaucracy that administers the CDBG Program. In some cases, CBOs can sponsor CDBG proposals and provide supportive public testimony. CBOs can administer CDBG activities. CBOs can also serve as watchdogs over cities' use of CDBG dollars to ensure that the money is used as intended, and CBOs can legally challenge a local government's use of its CDBG funds via administrative or court hearings (Dommel, 1984; Liebschutz, 1983; Orlebeke, 1983; Schmandt et al., 1983; Steger, 1984).

CBOs' roles relative to CDBGs vary from one community to another. In Chicago, CBOs made legal challenges to the city's use of CDBG funds by filing administrative complaints with the local HUD office. They charged that Chicago was not using CDBG funds to meet low-income housing requirements as stipulated in a previous court decision, and that the city was not making progress in implementing CDBG-funded rehabilitation programs and in achieving housing goals specified in Chicago's housing assistance program. The city did not make adequate provisions for all families that were displaced by urban renewal activities during the first three years of the CDBG program, nor had the city developed an adequate displacement plan, and furthermore, residents of a particular neighborhood objected to the city's designation of their neighborhood as a slum and as blighted. Although these challenges resulted in HUD's more intense review, monitoring, and placement of restrictions on Chicago's CDBG program, it did not result in Chicago losing any CDBG dollars (Orlebeke, 1983; Rich, 1993).

In contrast, CBOs in Rochester, New York, took a more cooperative approach with the local politicians relative to the distribution of CDBG funds. They worked directly with the local CDBG office to identify land use, planning needs, improvement strategies, and specific projects. As a result of this approach, Rochester avoided many of the contentious hearings that were often a critical part of the CDBG allocation process in other cities (Liebschutz, 1983).

Besides CBOs, individual citizens or informal groups of citizens might have input into the distribution of CDBG funds. Although HUD stipulated citizen participation in the CDBG program's original legislation and its 1978 amendment, the legislation did not stipulate the specific nature of that participation (Dommel and Associates, 1982; Rich, 1993). Because of these unclear guidelines, the type of citizen participation varies from locality to locality and remains more *advisory* than substantive. In Chicago, citizen participation was designed to allow citizens to comment on the city's CDBG application only at public hearings and to make written suggestions after it was ready for submittal to HUD (Rich, 1993).

In Milwaukee, the citizen participation plan was institutionalized through the creation of six neighborhood advisory councils (NACs) and a citywide citizen advisory committee (CAC). The NACs focused on the community and development needs of the neighborhoods they represented. NACs held public hearings on CDBG proposals. NACs could vote to fund, or not to fund a given proposal at any amount before the proposals proceeded to the other funding-decision levels (Gleiber and Steger, 1983; Steger, 1984). In contrast, the citizen advisory committee focused on citywide issues. The CAC reviewed all CDBG proposals submitted in a given year and made funding recommendations concerning the amount that should be allocated to those projects. Their impact on funding allocation decisions was, however, viewed as minimal (Steger, 1984). Both the NAC and CAC were eliminated in 1988 with the change of mayors in Milwaukee.

Although rules are meant to be guidelines for official decisions, the fairness and consistency in making such decisions, as it relates to CBOs representing various racial and ethnic groups, becomes a critical issue in many cities. Numerous studies suggest that some public bureaucracies' practices, policies, and procedures create a disadvantage for African-American neighborhoods and CBOs that are tantamount to institutional racism (Carmichael and Hamilton, 1967; Knowles and Prewitt, 1969; Thomas, 1986). This research will determine if Milwaukee's CDBG rules, which appeared race neutral, were applied fairly and consistently when CDBG allocation decisions were made.

Dozens of politicians, civil servants, CBOs, and informal citizen groups are involved in the decisions that allocate CDBG funds. Their exact role in a community changes over time and needs to be explored. Although this study will examine the effect of "who governs" on CDBG allocation and its impact on African-American neighborhoods, a vast research literature offers theoretical and empirical guidance in constructing an analysis.

Comparative studies of aggregate CDBG distribution data have found that some individual cities provided most of their CDBG dollars for low- and moderate-income areas. Cities such as Phoenix, Arizona, and Casa Grande, Arizona; Huntington Beach, California; and other communities were found to target a majority of their CDBG funds to low- and moderate-income communities (Dommel, 1980; Hall, 1982; Hall, 1983; Lovell, 1983; Rosenfeld, 1980; Sacco, 1982; Schmandt et al., 1983).

On the other hand, some cities spent the majority of their CDBG funds on projects that did not benefit low- and moderate-income areas by investing their CDBG funds in transitional areas facing decline. They used their CDBG funds to finance citywide public work projects, economic development projects, or to reward politically supported middle class neighborhoods (Ellison et al., 1986; Gleiber and Steger, 1983; Hall, 1983; Judd and Mushkatel, 1982; Liebschutz, 1983; Orlebeke, 1983; Peterson et al., 1986; Sacco, 1982; Schmandt et al., 1983; Wong and Peterson, 1986).

Researchers have studied the distribution of Milwaukee's CDBG funds. One study found that Milwaukee took a triage approach to allocating its CDBG funds between 1975 to 1981. The city used its CDBG funds to preserve the property-owner neighborhoods: those areas with high home ownership rates, located in the city's outer ring, and it used CDBG funds to support developmental projects. City government increased its share of CDBG funds allocated to those areas from 36 percent in 1979 to 60 percent in 1981. The city invested less than three percent of its CDBG funds in redistribution projects that benefited low- and moderate-income districts (Wong and Peterson, 1986). Other studies showed that Milwaukee used the majority of its CDBG funds to preserve its housing stock in transitional neighborhoods rather than low-income areas (Blumenfield, 1988; Peterson et al., 1986).

Another goal of these CDBG studies has been to determine if political or organizational models were the best predictor of allocation of 1979 CDBG funds to the neediest areas of Milwaukee. Steger (1984) found evidence that both the political and organizational models were useful in explaining and predicting how Milwaukee allocates its CDBG funds. A third approach to studying the distribution of CDBG funds in Milwaukee has been to determine whether federal guidelines, the city's priorities, or neighborhood preferences predicted CDBG distribution patterns. Again, using 1979 data, researchers found that the federal guidelines were the least responsive to community needs, followed by neighborhood CBOs, with the city's targeting mechanisms being the most responsive to community needs (Gleiber and Steger, 1983). Steger (1984) identified two factors that are rooted in the CDBG funding process: the ongoing, multiyear nature of some projects, and the year-to-year funding demands placed on the CDBG program. Ongoing CDBG-funded projects inhibit the discretion of local officials to allocate funding because they have already committed themselves to funding them. Because a commitment was made in another year to fund these projects, ongoing projects can circumvent rules and are insulated from political pressures. One would expect multiyear projects with a prior funding commitment to be funded (Steger, 1984).

Steger further stated that excessive requests for CDBG funding placed another constraint on the CDBG program. The monetary amounts requested in CDBG proposals are the demands to which the CDBG program must respond. Steger noted that in 1979 in Milwaukee, $42 million in CDBG requests were contained in the 153 proposals that were ultimately considered by the CDPC. Milwaukee's CDBG entitlement that year was approximately half that amount, or $21.4 million. Some proposals were rejected, and some were funded at less than the requested amount (Steger, 1984).

These studies on the CDBG program in Milwaukee were limited for several reasons. One weakness was that they studied CDBG allocations that took place under the same mayor, Henry Maier. Besides failing to take into account the variation created by the change in mayors, these studies are based on data collected before 1986. This research will update research on Milwaukee's CDBG program by studying it from 1975 to 1997, under two separate mayoral administrations. It will further consider the changes that occurred (a new mayor, new and sensitive common council members, increase in African-American elected officials, demographic changes) that affected the CDBG program during this time period. Moreover, this study focused on CDBG allocation patterns that occurred between 1975 to 1997 when the city used the same CDBG funding allocation process.

In 1997, the community block grant administration (CBGA) switched to a new CDBG allocation process for 1998 that made any CDBG comparison after 1997 to earlier years noncomparable. Finally, none of these studies addressed the role of race in the distribution of Milwaukee CDBG funds.

Because of the qualitative nature of this research, this study will not be "testing" these different explanations so much as using them as points of departure for understanding how CDBG funds were distributed in Milwaukee. The literature will be used as a guide rather than for proposing formal hypotheses for statistical analysis. Beyond this, the research goal was to understand the degree to which CDBG dollars were awarded by need, as the program rules specify, or by other considerations, such as race. By tracing the flow of decision making and investigating the decision making process, this study seeks to uncover the manner in which race has shaped this process in Milwaukee's CDBG program.

The CBGA office created by Council Resolution number 74-92 administers the city of Milwaukee's CDBG program. It is responsible for implementing, monitoring, and evaluating almost every aspect of the local CDBG program. This agency is under the control of the mayor, who appoints the CBGA director to serve at the chief executive's pleasure. The CBGA office also makes funding recommendations on all CDBG proposals considered in a given year and those recommendations are submitted to the Community Development Policy Committee (CDPC) (Community Block Grant Administration [CBGA], 1995; Gleiber and Steger, 1983).

Although the CBGA office administers the CDBG program, the CDPC, an advisory committee of the common council, makes policies and sets guidelines for the CDBG program. During this study period, the CDPC consisted of eight to ten members: the mayor or his or her designee; eight council members including the president of the council or his or her designee; and the city comptroller or his or her designee. The chairperson of the committee is the mayor, and the vice chair is the council president or his or her designee, who typically chairs the CDPC meetings. The CDPC provides policy direction to the CBGA in carrying out its responsibilities. It further reviews, rejects, or otherwise modifies the CBGA's recommendations regarding allocations to a particular project. The CDPC's funding decisions must be approved by the council and then signed by the mayor

(CBGA, 1995; Gleiber and Steger, 1983; Legislative Reference Bureau, 1994).

The awarding of CDBG funds in Milwaukee involved an extensive review process. It started with the development of its annual funding allocation plan (FAP), which outlined the city's policies on the CDBG program and the ten eligible program categories. HUD imposed funding caps on two of the ten funding categories, public services (15 percent) and administration (20 percent). Although HUD defined the general categories of CDBG-eligible activities and their caps, it did not define the specific activities or the funding allocation process that the city had to use (United States Department of Housing and Urban Development [HUD], 1996). The FAP was then given to the CDPC for its approval. After the CDPC approved the FAP, the CBGA developed the request for proposals (RFP) that was used as the CDBG application. CBOs and city agencies applied for CDBG funds in a particular program category via this RFP. After receiving the agencies' CDBG proposals, the CBGA staff evaluated them and made its CDBG recommendations in consultation with the mayor's office. The CBGA/mayor's office could change the requested amount. No scoring weights were given to CDBG proposals, nor were they ranked for funding purposes.

After the mayor/CBGA's office issued its CDBG recommendations, the mayor held public hearings on them over a two-day period to allow for comments. Those CDBG recommendations, along with a summary description of CBOs' proposals, performance records, and program descriptions were forwarded to the CDPC members in the CDBG briefing book, for their recommendations. Before making its CDBG recommendations, the CDPC held its own public hearings for CBOs to discuss their CDBG proposals. CDPC's CDBG recommendations were then forwarded to the zoning, neighborhoods, and development committee (ZN&D) or the finance and personnel committee (F&P), which could modify CDBG funding recommendations before they were forwarded to the full common council for its recommendations. The common council's CDBG recommendations were then forwarded to the mayor, who had to accept or veto them. If the mayor wanted to change the common council's CDBG recommendations, he had to veto an entire CDBG funding category, rather than modifying individual CDBG recommendations. He did not have line-item veto authority, nor could he veto a subcategory within a broader

CDBG category. The lawmakers could override the mayor's veto by a two-thirds vote of its members. If the council overrode the mayor's veto, then the common council's CDBG recommendations remained intact. If the common council did not override the mayor's veto, those vetoed categories were referred back to the common council's standing committees, which started the CDBG funding review cycle again.

Chapter 3

The Socioeconomic Status
of Milwaukee's African Americans

Similar to many older industrial cities, Milwaukee's total population declined in the 1980s and 1990s, falling from 669,014 people in
1975 to 628,088 people in 1990. Despite this overall decrease, the
city's African-American population grew markedly, from 123,683 in
1975 to 191,255 in 1990. The African-American population in Milwaukee increased from 18 percent of all residents in 1975 to 30.4 percent in 1990 (United States Department of Commerce, Bureau of
Census 1970, 1975, 1980, 1990). The city also lost a significant part
of its manufacturing base. During the late 1970s and 1980s, Milwaukee lost 27,500 high-paying manufacturing jobs while gaining 19,000
low-paying service jobs (Binkley and White, 1991). Such a loss of
manufacturing jobs has had a devastating impact on African-American communities throughout the United States (Gurda, 1999; Wilson,
1996).

In metropolitan Milwaukee, most African Americans lived in the
city of Milwaukee, a fact that did not change at all during the 1980s.
In 1980, 98.3 percent of metropolitan African Americans resided in
the city of Milwaukee with 97.8 percent living there in 1990 (Gilbert,
1991). Figures such as these were often cited to highlight the hypersegregation in Milwaukee, as African Americans showed very low
rates of suburbanization.

Milwaukee's African-American communities had some of the
highest poverty rates in the United States. In the 1970s, the poverty
rate in two of the city's predominantly African-American neighborhoods (Halyard Park, 37.3 percent and Garfield, 20.6 percent) was
more than two to four times higher than the city's poverty rate of 8.1
percent (Edari, 1977). Between 1980 and 1990, Milwaukee ranked
third out of fifty cities in the growth of extreme poverty census tracts

(40 percent of residents in the census tract lived below the poverty level) for African Americans. It ranked fifth in the number of poverty tracts; third in the number of distressed census tracts; and sixth in the number of severely distressed census tracts (Kasarda, 1993). Another study found that between 1980 and 1990 Milwaukee had the largest increase of ghetto poverty (defined as 40 percent of residents in a census tract living below the poverty level) in the nation. The rate among African Americans doubled between 1980 and 1990, increasing from 25.2 percent to 54.8 percent. The number of Milwaukee's African Americans living in poverty increased from 37,535 in 1980 to 107,482 in 1990, an increase of 69,947 individuals or 186 percent (Jargowsky, 1994).

Abramson and Tobin (1994) found that between 1980 and 1990, Milwaukee had the largest dissimilarity index of poor people (mostly African Americans) of any major city in the United States. Between 1980 and 1990, the index of dissimilarity for poor people in Milwaukee increased from 45.9 to 54.2. In absolute terms, the number of poor people increased from 89,345 in 1980 to 162,150 in 1990. Martin (1996) documented an increase in the poverty rate for African Americans in Milwaukee between 1980 and 1990. In 1980, twenty-five of the thirty-nine (65 percent) majority African-American census tracts (defined as 75 percent or greater African Americans) had more than 40 percent of their population living below the poverty level. By 1990, thirty-eight of forty-seven (82 percent) majority African-American census tracts had residents living in poverty. The mean census tract poverty rate for African Americans in Milwaukee increased from 35.6 percent in 1980 to 48.8 percent in 1990 (Martin, 1996).

The Wisconsin Council on Children and Families study revealed a dramatic increase in the number of African Americans living in ghetto poverty in the Milwaukee metropolitan area. It found that 25 percent of all African Americans in Milwaukee lived in ghetto poverty (census tracts where 40 percent or more of the residents live in poverty) in 1980, which doubled to 50 percent by 1990. The situation was even worse for African-American children. More than 60 percent of African-American children lived in ghetto poverty during this period (Wisconsin Council on Children and Families, 1994).

The bleak picture painted by the poverty statistics were borne out by data on recipients of Aid for Families with Dependent Children (AFDC). Rose (1992) found that the poverty population in Milwaukee grew by more than one-third between 1982 and 1988 for those families (mostly African Americans) receiving AFDC. Similarly, another study indicated that the percentage of African Americans receiving public assistance in the form of AFDC/general assistance increased from 36.5 percent in 1980 to 43.1 percent in 1990. The study found that in 1980, 93.6 percent of majority African-American census tracts (defined as 75 percent or greater African Americans) in the city were above the neighborhood distress level for receiving public assistance. A neighborhood was considered distressed when four of the seven distress indicators (poverty rate, male joblessness, public assistance usage, teen drop-out rate, female-headed families, labor force participation, and unemployment rate) were one standard deviation from the 1980 national mean. By 1990, this pattern had increased to 94.4 percent (Martin, 1996).

Although the data showed that poverty was widespread among Milwaukee's African Americans, recent trends indicate that the poverty situation might actually be getting worse. The 1994 elimination of Milwaukee County's General Assistance Program (GA), which provided public subsidies to unemployed males, contributed to the increased intensity of African-American poverty rate. When the program was terminated, 5,500 poor people in Milwaukee County were left without financial means. Over 80 percent of those males affected by the elimination of the general assistance program were African Americans and given the data on residential segregation, it is likely that most of them lived within the city of Milwaukee (Enriquez, 1995).

Despite having high poverty rates among its African-American population, Milwaukee consistently attracted poorer African Americans. A 1994 study of migration patterns of poor African Americans in the United States found that Milwaukee was one of the top ten destinations for them. Between 1985 and 1990, Milwaukee attracted 6,834 poor African Americans from other states (Frey, 1994; Murphy, 1994b).

In addition to having high poverty rates, Milwaukee's African Americans experienced some of the highest unemployment rates in the United States during this study period. In the 1970s, the unemployment rates for African-American males (8.3 percent) and African-American females (8.2 percent) were more than twice that of Caucasian males (3.5 percent) and Caucasian females (3.6 percent) in

Milwaukee (Edari, 1977). Between 1980 and 1986, the African-American unemployment rate increased from 13.9 percent to 25.9 percent, the highest unemployment rate of any racial group in Milwaukee (McNeely and Kinlow, 1987). A comparative study of 1985 unemployment rates in twenty-five major cities demonstrated high levels of both absolute and relative unemployment in Milwaukee's African-American community. In 1985, 27.9 percent of African Americans were unemployed, a rate second only to Detroit. The unemployment rate for Milwaukee's African Americans was 4.65 times higher than the unemployment rate of Milwaukee's Caucasians (Kole, 1987).

This high rate of unemployment for African Americans in Milwaukee during the 1980s continued throughout the 1990s. Martin (1996) noted that in majority African-American census tracts in Milwaukee, the unemployment rate increased from 16 percent in 1980 to 25.6 percent in 1990. In 1990, another study found that the first-quarter unemployment rate for young African-American men in Milwaukee was estimated at 60 percent (Rose et al., 1992). In 1992 the overall unemployment rate in the Milwaukee metropolitan area was 5 percent, yet African Americans' unemployment rate reached 23.9 percent (Nichols, 1993b). The unemployment rate for African Americans (22.7 percent) in metropolitan Milwaukee was the second highest in the country, exceeded only by the 27.9 percent rate that African Americans experienced in the Minneapolis-St. Paul area (Nichols, 1993a). In 1994, the unemployment rate disparity for African Americans in Milwaukee was the fourth highest among the nation's largest fifty communities (Comptroller's Office, 1996).

Milwaukee's African Americans live in one of the most racially segregated cities in the nation. Massey and Denton (1989) used five indicators to measure levels of segregation (evenness, exposure, clustering, centralization, and concentration) for the nation's largest metropolitan areas. They found Milwaukee to be one of six cities (Baltimore, Chicago, Cleveland, Detroit, and Philadelphia) to have high segregation scores on all five of these measures. They termed these communities "hypersegregated" (Massey and Denton, 1989). In 1986, Milwaukee was ranked first of the largest fifty cities in the percentage of African Americans living in racially segregated neighborhoods. Approximately 97.5 percent of African Americans in Milwaukee lived in racially segregated neighborhoods (McNeely and Kinlow, 1987).

The racial segregation of African Americans in Milwaukee continued into the 1990s. The 1990 United States census revealed that Milwaukee was the fourth most racially segregated city in America behind Gary, Indiana, Cleveland, Ohio, and Chicago, Illinois (Holt, 1994; Tuerina, 1993). Milwaukee had the fifth highest African Americans to Caucasian segregation index of 83.9. Only Detroit (86.7); Cleveland (87.5); Chicago (87.8); and Gary (90.6) exceeded this segregation index (Massey and Denton, 1993).

Milwaukee's racial segregation contributed to high isolation rates between the city's African Americans and Caucasians. High isolation areas were defined as areas with at least 90 percent African-American residents. In 1980, Milwaukee ranked tenth among the nation's fifty largest areas in the isolation of African Americans with an isolation index of 69.5. In the 1990s, Milwaukee ranked twelfth out of the nation's fifty largest metropolitan areas in the isolation of African Americans. In 1990, 42 percent of all Milwaukee's African Americans lived in isolation (Yinger, 1995).

Housing realtors and insurance companies have limited the ability of African Americans to move out of segregated neighborhoods in Milwaukee. Housing realtors were found to have steered African Americans in Milwaukee away from nonminority areas when they were searching to purchase a home. Yinger (1995) cited a study that monitored the advertisement practices of one of the largest real estate companies in Milwaukee over a three-year period. The study found that the property listings in largely African-American and integrated neighborhoods were only half as likely to be advertised in the *Milwaukee Journal,* and only one-fourth were as likely to have an open house in comparison to listings in Caucasian neighborhoods (Yinger, 1995). Similarly, Squires (1994) indicated that housing testing programs conducted by the Metropolitan Milwaukee Fair Housing Council routinely discovered that realtors were steering African Americans away from properties in majority Caucasian neighborhoods.

In addition to racial steering by realtors, insurance companies redlined African-American communities, thus limiting their ability to obtain mortgage insurance. Squires and Velez (1987) found that insurance companies were more likely to issue regular insurance policies in majority Caucasian communities as compared to African-American neighborhoods. They found that minority composition of the zip code area was the variable that best correlated with voluntary market insurance. As minority concentration increased, the amount of voluntary market insurance being written decreased (Squires and Velez, 1987). This insurance redlining practice has been estimated to have cost African Americans in Milwaukee more than $1.9 billion in lost assets resulting from their inability to purchase homes (Madison and Squires, 1996).

Considerable evidence exists which indicates that Milwaukee's African Americans with comparable incomes were less likely to receive loans from financial institutions than other racial groups during this study period. Between 1983 and 1988, African Americans were rejected for loans 24.2 percent of the time compared to 6.2 percent for Caucasians. In almost all income categories, African Americans in Milwaukee were almost four times as likely to be rejected for loans as were Caucasians (Dedman, 1989).

African Americans' high loan rejection rates continued into the 1990s. In 1992, minorities were denied loans 19.8 percent of the time compared to 5.6 percent for Caucasians. Similarly, African Americans received less than 5 percent of home purchase loans despite accounting for 14 percent of Milwaukee's metropolitan population (Squires, 1993). In 1993, minority applicants were denied loans 22.3 percent of the time compared to Caucasians who were denied loans 6.6 percent of the time for a 3.4 loan rejection disparity rate. This rejection rate was the highest among the nation's fifty largest metropolitan areas (Gilmer, 1995; Held, 1995; Norman, 1993). In 1994, Milwaukee continued to have the highest racial disparities in loan rejection rates in the nation. Minority applicants were rejected for loans 3.7 times more than Caucasian applicants (Comptroller's Office, 1996). Still in 1994, minority applicants were six times more likely to be rejected for loans based on their credit history than were Caucasians (Comptroller's Office, 1996). Thus, one in every three African Americans was rejected for loans, compared to one in every thirteen Caucasian applicants (Norman, 1996b).

African Americans' credit problems existed regardless of income levels. Minority applicants with income between $46,000 to $55,680 were rejected for loans six times more often than Caucasians with similar income. Even worse, minority loan applicants with income over $55,680 were 9.25 more likely to be denied a loan than Caucasians with similar incomes. In contrast, minorities with incomes under $37,120 were 3.55 times more likely to be denied a loan than their Caucasian counterparts (Comptroller's Office, 1996). Thus, minorities with higher income levels were more likely to be rejected for loans when compared to Caucasians.

The situation did not get better as financial institutions left Milwaukee's African-American neighborhoods. In 1994, Milwaukee ranked as one of the worst cities for having banking facilities located in mostly Caucasian areas versus African-American neighborhoods. Milwaukee tied five other cities with having the thirteenth worst ratio of banking facilities located in Caucasian neighborhoods versus those in African-American neighborhoods ("Bank access limited," 1995). Instead, a number of check-cashing businesses and payday loan stores that charged high fees and interest rates opened in the city's African-American communities (Squires and O'Connor, 1998).

Income for African Americans in Milwaukee also fared poorly during this study period. In 1984, African Americans' median household income was $10,000 per year. This amount was 48 percent of Caucasians' household income in Milwaukee (McNeely and Kinlow, 1987). Another study found that among the forty-eight largest standard metropolitan statistical areas (SMSAs) with an African-American population of more than 100,000, African Americans in Milwaukee trailed all but Buffalo and Newark on nine economic measures: home ownership, value of homes, income, and other indicators (O'Hare, 1986; Rummler, 1986). By 1994, African Americans in Milwaukee had the highest racial income disparity among the nation's fifty largest metropolitan areas (Comptroller's Office, 1996; "Income gap widens," 1995).

The relative low values of Milwaukee's African-American homes further reflected their disadvantaged economic status. In 1980, African Americans in Milwaukee had the lowest home value of any racial/ethnic group in the city. African Americans' average home value for an owner-occupied home was $28,500, compared to $34,600 for Hispanics, $34,700 for Native Americans, $47,000 for Caucasians, and $50,000 for Asians (McNeely and Kinlow, 1987). This pattern continued throughout the 1980s. In 1988, 21 percent of single-family homes in Milwaukee were valued at less than $35,000. However, in predominantly African-American neighborhoods, 78 percent of single-family homes were valued at less than $35,000 (Squires, 1994).

Another analysis showed that houses in predominantly Caucasian areas purchased in the 1970s increased in value by 300 percent in the 1990s, whereas comparable houses purchased in predominantly African-American neighborhoods declined during the same time period (Nichols, 1995a).

While African Americans were having difficulty obtaining mortgage loans, the availability of low-income housing in the African-American communities was decreasing due to demolition. "Within the boundaries of Holton to N. 35th streets, and W. Keefe Ave. to W. Walnut St., 3,314 housing units were demolished from 1990 through 1997. Only 185 new units were built" (Norman and Borowski, 1999, p. A1).

Milwaukee's African Americans did not benefit much from the major revitalization projects in the city's central business district (CBD). During the 1980s and 1990s, Milwaukee's primary approach to revitalizing the city was the development of its CBD. Although the city spent millions of tax dollars on these projects, the city's African Americans did not receive many of the intended spin-offs. Of all the new employees hired in firms created after 1982 in the CBD, African Americans received only 7.4 percent of those jobs. Caucasians received 88 percent of those jobs (Levine and Zipp, 1994).

Furthermore, African Americans did not receive a significant share of the upper management or professional level jobs, further limiting their economic chances. "Of all African Americans and Latinos working in post to 1982 firms downtown in 1992, only 3.4 percent held managerial positions" (Levine and Zipp, 1994, p. 11). Others have documented the lack of African Americans in professional and managerial positions. In 1992, data from the U.S. Equal Employment Opportunity Commission (EEOC) in metropolitan Milwaukee found that African Americans held just 2.8 percent of official and managerial positions and 3.3 percent of professional positions. This was lower than the national average of 5.2 percent for officials and managers, and 5.5 percent for professionals (Joshi, 1994). In 1994, African Americans held 17.1 percent of all managerial or professional positions in the local government of Milwaukee. This was a decrease from 1993 when African Americans held 19.5 percent of professional and managerial positions (Johnson-Elie, 1996).

The likelihood of more African Americans moving into these managerial and professional positions was unlikely. Many African-

American professionals were leaving Milwaukee because of a lack of career opportunities, and African-American professionals from other cities were not migrating to Milwaukee for jobs (Frey, 1994; Johnson-Elie, 1996; Joshi, 1994; Murphy, 1994a).

African Americans were not receiving their share of high-paying professional and managerial positions from the city's major redevelopment projects or from private businesses. They were instead receiving a disproportionate share of the lower-paying jobs. Levine and Zipp (1994) noted that among all employees making $40,000 annually in CBD firms that started after 1982, African Americans and Latinos received 1.7 percent of those positions. By contrast, 22.7 percent of African Americans and Latinos earned under $10,000 in those firms and 16.1 percent of them made between $10,000 and $20,000 a year. In summary, 94.8 percent of all African Americans and Latinos earned under $20,000 in those firms compared to 43 percent of Caucasians who earned under $20,000 in those firms (Levine and Zipp, 1994).

Other researchers have documented the high concentration of African Americans in low paying jobs in Milwaukee. Rose et al. (1992) found that less than 3 percent of African Americans in their study were employed in government, construction, finance, realty, or insurance fields. Meanwhile, 90 percent of the jobs held by African Americans were in retail, day labor, and service-related jobs, which were generally the lowest paid positions.

Several consultant studies found that Milwaukee's African Americans have suffered because minority-owned businesses, which could have contributed to their economic well-being, have struggled to become established and to participate in the city's marketplace. In 1990, one study found that African Americans were underrepresented in the number of employees working in the skilled trades and construction fields. In 1981, African Americans accounted for only 1.4 percent of the employees in construction and skilled crafts. Between 1980 and 1988, only seventy-nine (7.9 percent) of the 990 apprenticeship positions for trade unions went to racial minorities despite a goal of 12.5 percent for those groups (Conta and Associates Inc., 1990). Finally, the study cited considerable anecdotal evidence revealing that African-American businesses were excluded from the business market by pervasive discrimination and a hostile racial environment. A later minority business disparity study provided statistical and anecdotal evidence of racial discrimination against African-American businesses in Milwaukee (Affirmative Action Consulting LTD., Moore, and Associates, 1992).

These aforementioned conditions have had devastating impacts on the socioeconomic status of the city's African Americans as reflected in their wide range of social problems (drug abuse, broken families, poor housing quality, crime, hopelessness, unemployment, homelessness, homicides, poverty). These conditions showed that African-American neighborhoods were in desperate need of a major infusion of resources or control over resources such as CDBG to address these problems. The CDBG program provides one source of potential funds for addressing these problems. Although the CDBG program cannot solve all of the problems facing Milwaukee's African-American neighborhoods, it can fund programs specifically designed to address some of these problems.

Chapter 4

Surveying the Impact of Race in Milwaukee's Allocation of CDBG Funds

What role does race play in the distribution of CDBG funds? Respondents to the researcher-initiated mail surveys and interviews offered different opinions. Despite the wide variety of individuals asked to participate in the survey, their answers came in three general groupings. Many respondents answered that race does play a role in that CDBG funds are more liberally distributed to African-American controlled CBO's or organizations that are established to improve the quality of life for African Americans living in segregated neighborhoods. The second grouping of responses stated that race does not play a role and that the city of Milwaukee has succeeded in its effort to allocate CDBG funds in a race-neutral manner. Finally, a third group stated that it believed that African Americans are not getting their fair share of CDBG funds.

In the first grouping, respondents suggested that African-American CBOs and African-American districts receive more funds than Caucasian CBOs and Caucasian districts. These answers reflected a perception among many in Milwaukee that CDBG programs and funds were part of a transfer payment system that targeted non-Caucasians living in poverty or in poor areas. Although one CBO representative stated, "Odds are the more African-American the organization, the more likely funds [CDBG] will be less, compared to comparable organizations," other CBO representatives expressed the opposite sentiment, as in the following statement: "It seems, although I have not seen the data on this, that high need areas that get the public service dollars are African-American communities." Some observers noted that if African Americans controlled the CBO, it would receive the requested level of CDBG dollars. These perspectives portray a widespread sentiment that many residents of metropolitan Milwaukee believed—that race did play a role in the distribution of CDBG funds—and that African Americans benefited.

A second viewpoint suggested that race did not play a role in the distribution of CDBG funds. Instead, the distribution of CDBG funds was race neutral. As one CBO representative stated, "I do not think distribution of CDBG funds has to do with racial composition of a community." Another CBO director stated that there is a strong effort to balance the CDBG funds racially, across different racial areas of the city. One CBO leader noted, "I believe CBGA is fair in utilizing its funding. Milwaukee is a racially segregated city and CDBG tries to address that problem." Finally, another CBO leader made a similar observation, "I believe significant efforts are made to ensure that all areas in the CDBG target areas are served regardless of racial composition."

A third perspective claimed that African Americans were at a disadvantage in the allocation of CDBG funds. Proponents of this viewpoint cited the defunding and differential treatment of African-American agencies, allocation patterns, and other actions as evidence that African Americans were at a disadvantage in the distribution of CDBG funds.

As the three different groupings of respondents show, many residents of metropolitan Milwaukee believe that race does indeed play a role in the allocation of the CDBG funds. But there is no agreement as to whether this impact causes African Americans to receive preferential treatment or adverse treatment. Though some respondents contend that the CDBG allocation process is race neutral, other respondents provide convincing evidence of the opposite: in Milwaukee's CDBG allocation process, race plays a significant role in determining levels of funding and which CBOs have received CDBG funds.

To fully examine this evidence and analyze its significance, this chapter will examine two perspectives highlighted by the respondents: (1) It will focus on the claim that African Americans were favored, and (2) it will investigate the claim that African Americans were denied a fair share.

For many of the respondents claiming that African Americans received preferential treatment, their position was based on the racial composition of neighborhoods within the CDBG boundaries, the racial composition of CBOs that received CDBG funds, and the racial composition of the CDPC—the city-sponsored committee that formally advised and commented upon all applications for funding.

These respondents claimed that the neighborhoods within CDBG boundaries where CDBG funds were directed contained mostly racial minorities (African Americans and Hispanics). As one African-American public official stated, race plays a role only to the extent that the CDBG target area was heavily concentrated with African Americans. Another Caucasian public official echoed a similar point. He stated that most CDBG funds were allocated to areas in which "people of color" (African Americans and Hispanics) lived. Several other public officials indicated that although CDBG funds were not specifically earmarked to benefit people of color, people of color were concentrated in Milwaukee's poorest areas that received CDBG funds. One Caucasian public official stated, "Race plays a role only, in my estimation, that HUD requires that the bulk of the funds be allocated for low-income and moderate-income areas, which for the most part are minorities, who are the primary beneficiaries."

Milwaukee's CBGA requirement to look at the composition of a CBO's board of directors suggested that race actually played a positive role in the distribution of CDBG funds to the African-American community and CBOs. As one Caucasian public official notes, "The Community Block Grant Administration (CBGA) seeks to fund CBOs that are representative of the community [African Americans and Hispanics]." He stated, "While there is a role that race plays, part of our goal is to try to empower minority agencies [those whose boards are reflective of the neighborhood areas] and give them money. The agencies that receive funds reflect the population of the community." Another African-American public official agreed. He suggested, that at the request of the CDPC, a breakdown of representation of African Americans on CBOs' board of directors and staff be included in its reviews of CDBG proposals. The CBGA considered such representation as it made CDBG funding decisions.

This line of reasoning suggested that the CBGA office was conscious of the representation of African Americans on CBOs' board of directors and staff when it made funding decisions. Although the CBGA required CBOs to provide this information, interviews, survey responses, and an extensive review of public records showed that racial compositions of boards of directors and staff did not influence the common council's or CBGA/mayor's decision to fund an agency.

No proof existed that indicated CDBG funds were denied, reduced, increased, or withheld from any agency because of the racial composition of its board of directors or staff. Without evidence of CDBG funding decisions being impacted as a result of the racial composition of boards or staff, it is reasonable to suggest that the CBO director's report was gathered for informational purposes only.

In addition to the geographical location of the CDBG boundaries and the makeup of CBOs' board of directors, this group of respondents claimed, the representation of African Americans on the CDPC suggested that they would get more CDBG funds for their neighborhoods. African Americans were well represented on the CDPC during this study period. In 1995, African Americans made up 40 percent of the CDPC members (four of ten members). This level of representation has been almost consistent throughout the CDBG program's history. African Americans accounted for approximately one-third (two to four members) of the seven to ten members on the CDPC during most of this study period. As one Caucasian city councilor stated, "Race isn't a negative factor in the distribution of CDBG funds because you have African Americans making such decisions. If you look at the composition of the CDPC, African Americans are adequately represented. You have at least three minority people on the CDA making allocation decisions."

This point reflected a number of erroneous assumptions about how the city's CDBG process worked. One, it suggested that the number of African-American councilors on the CDPC was adequate to ensure that CDBG funds were going to African-American communities. Three of seven (or four of ten) remains a minority-voting bloc. This perspective assumed that those African-American councilors were voting as a bloc along racial lines to fund the same CDBG projects, which was not the case. In reality, African Americans reflected a significant minority of the votes on the CDPC. If and when they acted as a solid bloc, they still needed to win Caucasian votes to form a majority. Without a coalition that crossed racial lines, African-American councilors could not use the CDPC to formally endorse any CDBG project. On the other hand, a majority of Caucasian councilors could and have voted as a bloc against the African-American minority when making CDBG allocation decisions. When African-American councilors were successful in building a multiracial coalition in the CDPC, their chances of winning a favorable recommendation from the full common council diminished in terms of probability and number of votes. When the full common council took up the CDBG allocation decisions, the African-American representation dropped from 40 percent to 30 percent.

To those who claimed that the racial composition of CBOs and their geographical location in African-American neighborhoods helped African Americans win preferential treatment, the hard data presented a different picture. In many African-American neighborhoods, African-American CBOs closed their doors and went out of business. As one government official stated, "In many cases, funding for a given aldermanic district will be limited if there is a lack of competent qualified agencies who are headquartered in those districts." He further stated that if viable CBOs were not located in African-American communities, those areas would receive less CDBG funding. If this were the case, he pointed out, then CDBG funding would go to CBOs located outside those areas.

As one CBO representative stated, "I believe that the racial composition is less important than whether there is an active CBO in the area requesting funds or an active alderperson securing funds for an area." Similarly, one Caucasian public official stated, there were African-American neighborhoods that were not covered by a CBO, which made it harder for the council to allot CDBG funds to an African-American CBO that operated within an African-American council district. Milwaukee had only one remaining African-American housing rehabilitation CBO, which represented the largest CDBG-funded category. This made it harder for African-American districts and African-American CBOs to receive a greater share of CDBG funding. An African-American public official echoed this viewpoint. He stated that although there were some strong CBOs in parts of the African-American community, in other parts there were no CBOs located to fund. The weak representation of CBOs in African-American neighborhoods got worse. In 1994, within some of the poorest areas of African-American neighborhoods, several CBOs went out of business. According to one respondent, the absence of African-American CBOs between 35th Street to 1st Street, and Center Street to North Avenue make it impossible for a neighborhood-controlled CBO to receive CDBG funds for that area.

The other perspective offered by survey respondents revolved around the claim that race negatively influenced the distribution of

CDBG funds to African-American areas and CBOs. Although the preceding discussion indicated that some CBOs believed that the African-American community did not get shortchanged with the CDBG program, others believed it did. To some respondents, race appeared to be a major factor in the evaluation of CDBG projects in several areas. The decision to take away a CBO's CDBG funding was one such issue. When the city government enacted this decision, it generated loudly aired allegations of racism and created a number of racial disputes. Throughout the debate and in their responses to the survey that is part of this research, respondents claimed that African-American CBOs appeared more likely to have their CDBG funding eliminated or to be given restrictions than Caucasian CBOs. Numerous examples were provided that showed that the termination of CDBG funding appeared to be racially motivated. Some respondents believed African-American CBOs were held to higher performance standards than Caucasian CBOs.

Respondents noted that many of their claims of race playing a negative role could be seen in the decision to eliminate funding for one African-American CBO, North Division Resident Association. In announcing this decision, the city government formally claimed that North Division Resident Association did not meet its performance goals. Located in one of the poorest areas of the city, it served a predominantly African-American community. This agency had completed less than half of its contracted housing goals, even after program restrictions were placed on the agency. This agency was accused of misappropriating CDBG funds and not serving the intended population. As a result of these charges, it lost its CDBG funding.

Supporters of this agency believed that the elimination of its CDBG funding was racially motivated and that it was accomplished as follows. One representative of a CBO stated bluntly,

> North Division was slandered and killed by the Mayor because they did not acquiesce to the party line. This is done by the monitoring staff, nickeling and diming each piece of paper work a group submits for expenditures. This then creates problems regarding withholding taxes, suppliers, and staff salaries.

This person believed that race was the motivating factor for putting these restrictions on the agency. Once North Division lost its CDBG funds, its capacity to carry out another major inner-city housing initiative, Genesis, was limited. It did not have the funding to pay for administrative staff to carry out other projects. This agency lost its CDBG funding and eventually went out of business.

Besides the restrictions being placed on African-American CBOs, those groups were more likely to be denied funding for new initiatives. This point was illustrated by the denial of funding to Genesis, the African-American CBO initiative previously mentioned. North Division Resident Association wanted to construct new houses for low- and moderate-income people in Milwaukee's central city, a deviation from the city's triage policy of rehabilitating properties. The project would have been located in the heart of Milwaukee's African-American community (Teutonia Avenue and North Avenue). Several issues were disputed. One issue centered on the per-unit housing cost of the proposed project. The housing units were considered too costly to do on a public scale and required more city funds than originally anticipated.

Furthermore, the environmental cost of cleaning up the proposed site for the project was another point of contention. The proposed project site had some contamination problems that needed to be removed and the site cleanup would have added significant costs to the project. According to one African-American elected official, several public officials expressed major concerns regarding those costs, contributing to its denial of funds. Likewise, there were political clashes contributing to the defeat of this housing initiative. Representatives of North Division were involved in personality conflicts and philosophical disagreements with the CBGA/mayor's office. These differences helped contribute to the denial of funding for the agency, and Genesis was not developed.

The denial of funding for the project would have other implications according to one African-American public official. It prevented a new approach from being developed by an African-American CBO, which was consistent with HUD's intended use of CDBG funds. The CBO was "constructing," rather than rehabilitating, low-income housing units for residents in the heart of the central city, which was unprecedented. Genesis would have provided employment opportunities for many African-American professionals to develop a major housing project. Such experience would have provided the African-American community with professionally trained individuals with expertise in the construction of low-income housing. The project would have enabled North Division to build equity from that initiative to undertake other major development efforts. When Genesis was not funded, the project and the potential benefits were lost. The proposed site remained as a large vacant lot and a sore spot in the African-American community for several years after this project was defeated.

The elimination of funding for African-American CBOs was illustrated by another example. One African-American CBO, which was an advocate for minority businesses, lost its CDBG funding due to some concerns about the agency's fiscal practices. The agency, which had received $50,000 a year, had its funding cut to one dollar, which kept an account open for a year. The following year, that account was closed, resulting in the elimination of funding for that CBO.

In addition to having their CDBG funding eliminated and new funding denied, African-American CBOs were more likely to have program and financial restrictions placed on them by the CBGA than Caucasian CBOs. The O. C. White Soul Club was charged with mismanagement of funds, hiring the spouse of the agency's executive director, and not meeting housing rehabilitation goals. CBGA placed contingencies on that agency as a condition for it receiving CDBG funds. The agency was informed that it needed to reform or risk losing its CDBG funding. The CBO was given technical assistance and was provided CDBG funds, but funding was eliminated a year later.

Another African-American CBO, Project Respect, had restrictions placed on its funding. This CBO was involved in crime prevention efforts, youth recreation, block club activities, and other social programs. It had ties to an African-American militia group that advocated violence. An African-American former alderman was the leader of the African-American militia. The CBGA wanted to cut the agency's CDBG funding, but the local HUD agency intervened. HUD stated that the city could not cut the CBO's funding for association with the militia, but it could place the following restrictions on the agency:

- Supplies and equipment funded with CDBG dollars could not be used for the militia.
- The agency's staff could not perform militia activities during their regular work hours that were paid for with CDBG funds.
- The agency could not lease space from the militia using CDBG funds.

The CBGA placed these restrictions on the agency as a condition for it receiving CDBG dollars. As a result of those restrictions, Project Respect broke its visible ties from the African-American militia, and moved its office.

According to one respondent, another African-American CBO faced more restrictions than Caucasian CBOs. The Inner City Redevelopment Corporation (ICRC) worked to redevelop the inner city's major business strip. Its $90,000 CDBG request was held at the zoning, neighborhoods, and development committee (ZN&D), even though other CDBG projects were allowed to proceed through the CDBG review cycle. ICRC had "philosophical differences" with the mayor on several issues. One African-American public official indicated that this was the first time in the history of the CDBG program that a CBO's funding was taken out of the CDPC's recommendations at the ZN&D. The respondent indicated that a representative of this agency later met with a representative of the mayor's office and resolved its differences. This CBO was then provided CDBG dollars.

Although some of these African-American CBOs had some notable problems, it appeared that Caucasian CBOs with similar or worse problems were not penalized. One Caucasian economic development and housing CBO, Northwest Side Community Development Corporation (NWSCDC), was alleged to have misallocated CDBG funds. This CBO, located in a predominantly African-American area, could not account for thousands of its CDBG dollars. As one African-American activist stated, the agency disclosed accounting irregularities in its operations, which resulted in unpaid tax bills ($89,000), and also made incorrect reports to city officials. A copy of a funding and expenditure summary report by the agency revealed that it purchased a $3,000 insurance policy for a mobile watch program. The program's supervisor said there was no insurance for it.

The agency's questionable financial practices created other problems. The lack of money caused the agency to be delinquent on many accounts—a fact that generated considerable publicity in the local media. As one representative from an inner-city CBO stated

> The Northwest Side CDC this year was found to not have paid their bills including taxes ($185,000 plus), etc. However, no one in city hall including the mayor or his "alderman" made an issue of it and the agency was funded without major embarrassments.

Despite this report of substantial misconduct, NWSCDC was not defunded nor given program restrictions by the CBGA. Instead, this agency received $200,000 in new CDBG funds. Only one public official opposed its funding and voted against it.

This was consistent with another Caucasian housing CBO, Westside Conservation Corporation (WCC). It had purchased over 100 properties from the city with the promise of rehabilitating them. After several years, the agency did not have funds available to repair houses as stated in its CDBG contract. Yet the agency was not given any significant penalty. As one Caucasian councilor stated, "That agency was given a slap on the wrist. It didn't lose any funding, nor were restrictions placed on that agency by the CBGA Program." An African-American CDBG monitor confirmed this story. He stated that, "the CBO had a cash-flow problem, but it was one of our better performing CBOs, so we didn't penalize it."

In a similar instance, a newly funded Caucasian CBO, Milwaukee Housing Assistance Corporation (MHAC) was given CDBG funds to perform housing rehabilitation. Despite receiving CDBG funding for several years, it did not complete any properties. It was never defunded, penalized, nor threatened with a reduction of its allotment.

After examining the internal administration of CDBG funds for city agencies it can be concluded that racial considerations negatively influenced the distribution of CDBG funds. As one African-American former public official noted

> Race played a role that on the community level, most of the participants were minority residents. They lived in the targeted area. But as you move up in the [city's] decision-making processes (comptroller's office, DCD, RACM, etc.) the decision-making processes were [controlled] mostly by Caucasians.

A Caucasian former elected official echoed this point. She stated it more bluntly, "Race plays an unsubtle role in that most people that manage [CDBG] funds are Caucasian males. City-directed dollars to city agencies [Department of City Development (DCD); Community Development Administration (CDA), etc.] are directed by white males." Some support for these claims is cited in Table 4.1. It shows that the majority of city positions funded by CDBG dollars were held by Caucasians. Of the 219 city positions of which portions were paid by CDBG funds, Caucasians held 147 (67.4 percent); African Ameri-

TABLE 4.1. CDBG-Funded City Jobs, 1996 to 1997

City Agencies	CBO's Race			
	AA	**C**	**O**	**T**
CBGA	8	5	2	15
City Clerk	1	0	0	1
DCD	36	128	14	178
RACM	3	11	2	16
Comptroller	3	3	3	9
T	51	147	21	219

Source: CBGA, 1996a

AA = African Americans; C = Caucasians; O = Others; T = Total

cans held fifty-one (22.9 percent); and other racial groups held twenty-one (9.6 percent) of the positions.

An analysis of CDBG proposals showed that in the Department of City Development (DCD), which received millions of CDBG dollars annually, the CDBG staffing levels greatly exceeded the level of CDBG-funded activities. There were a number of individuals listed as being paid by CDBG funds, but they were not doing CDBG work based on the amount of work cited in their proposals and their job titles. Some of these positions would have been more appropriately funded by the city's tax-levy budget. CDBG funds were used to cover other city positions held by Caucasians, even when the persons were not doing CDBG-related work.

A large percentage of CDBG funds was awarded to city agencies. One African-American public official estimated that city agencies, which were overwhelmingly managed by Caucasian appointees of Mayor Norquist, received more than 50 percent of CDBG funds as of 1994. These agencies used CDBG dollars for hiring staff, purchasing services and equipment, and subcontracting purposes. Yet these decisions were made with little public review or input from the CDBG residents.

Besides situations that overtly pitted African Americans against Caucasians, the negative impact of race on the distribution of CDBG funds was subtle and often buried in the minutia of city government operations. CDBG funds were used to finance tax-levy services in

African-American neighborhoods throughout the 1970s and mid-1980s. Several former elected Caucasian and African-American officials noted that Milwaukee used a large share of CDBG funds to pay for regularly scheduled capital improvement projects (CIP) in the CDBG area in place of tax-levy dollars. As one Caucasian former alderwoman and one African-American former public official stated, the city decreased the amount of CDBG funds available to African-American CBOs by using a large portion of these funds to pay for capital improvement projects that had a citywide reach. One African-American city councilor said,

> One of the constant fights [against Mayor Maier] was for projects located in the CDBG area that empowered CBOs versus those projects that replaced tax dollars (streets, lights, sidewalks). CIPs were normally done by tax-levy dollars. This money [CDBG funds] was used outside of areas, which consisted mostly of African-Americans. CDBG funds were used as replacement for tax dollars instead of supplementing them.

The use of CDBG funds to pay for some tax-levy CIPs had several major impacts. It freed up tax-levy dollars for other capital improvement projects and other activities in mostly Caucasian areas outside the CDBG boundaries, and it reduced the total amount of CDBG dollars available to the African-American community. This decision diluted the impact of CDBG funds from neighborhood-specific to citywide projects. Likewise, the use of CDBG funds for CIPs in place of tax-levy funds actually became a subsidy for CIPs in Caucasian neighborhoods located outside the CDBG boundaries. By using CDBG funds in this manner, the city government in essence diverted funds from poorer neighborhoods into richer areas. As a result of this extra influx of funds, many Caucasian neighborhoods outside of the CDBG boundaries were able to take advantage of "freed up" tax-levy dollars that suddenly became available for other services and construction projects. As one council member noted about the tenure of Mayor Maier,

> the overwhelming majority of CDBG funds were being used for capital improvement projects. While CDBG funds were being used to fund capital projects in the CDBG area, other city funds

that had been scheduled to perform those projects were being used outside the CDBG boundaries.

Still, the use of CDBG dollars in place of tax-levy dollars had a major positive impact on the tax-paying residents of Milwaukee. It enabled the city to lower its tax rate because it was shifting tax-related functions to CDBG dollars. Finally, the use of CDBG dollars for CIPs kept those funds and jobs in city agencies, instead of being used for community programs.

This diversion of CDBG funds into CIPs forced African-American neighborhoods and CBOs to compete for a decreasing share of CDBG funds. As other racial minority groups (Asians, Native Americans, and Hispanics) grew and became politically active, they too were seeking CDBG funds to address socioeconomic problems in their communities. As one Caucasian public official noted,

> The share of CDBG funds going to African-American neighborhoods is decreasing because other groups (Hispanics, Asians) are more active and getting organized. These groups are seeking a piece of the CDBG pie and CDBG boundaries have been changed to include neighborhoods inhabited by those groups.

CBO requests (fiscal year 1995) for CDBG funds revealed that other minority groups were seeking CDBG funds more than ever. A listing of CBOs seeking CDBGs showed that the following types of agencies were seeking CDBG dollars: Hmong/American Friendship Association, Milwaukee Indian Economic Development Agency, Southeast Asian Youth Project, Hmong Pheng Housing, Tejauma Na Nia, Hispanic Chamber of Commerce, Latino Club, and Southeast Asian Business and Economic Development Project.

This chapter has shown that prominent Caucasian and African-American public officials believed that the structure of the CDBG program and the distribution of its funds had both benefits and drawbacks for the African-American community. Yet the benefits seemed to be more symbolic in nature and they had less severe consequences than the drawbacks. The positive impacts included defining the CDBG boundaries where a majority of African Americans lived in the city, including the number of African Americans serving on the CDPC, and examining the composition of CBOs' board of directors and staff when reviewing CDBG applications. For these reasons, it appeared that the African-American neighborhoods and CBOs were not at a disadvantage in the distribution of CDBG funds. They were well represented on the CDPC, and a majority of African Americans lived within the CDBG boundaries. Moreover, African-American common council members served on the CDPC, and they represented their interests. The mere presence of African-American common council members on the CDPC did not ensure that those areas received CDBG funds, especially when those members were a voting minority or did not vote along racial lines.

Similarly, the CBGA's examination of CDBG proposals to determine their board of directors' composition was symbolic. Although the CBGA office required CBOs to provide information on the racial composition of their board of directors and their staff, it has been asserted that these data influenced CDBG funding decisions. The CBGA did not reject or reduce funding to a CBO based solely on its level of representation of African Americans. The CBGA did not provide any threshold number for what level of representation it deemed sufficient for an agency to be considered representative of a community. To this end, this reporting requirement appeared to wield very little influence in the distribution of CDBG funds.

Finally, defining the CDBG boundaries to include a large segment of the African-American community did not ensure that African-American CBOs received those CDBG funds. Although on the surface a significant number of respondents believed that CDBG funds were going to predominantly African-American neighborhoods, many Caucasian CBOs located in those areas received the money. Any analysis of CDBG allocations to geographic areas should look beyond the aggregate dollar amount going to those areas and determine which specific racial groups (Caucasians, African Americans, etc.) within neighborhoods were actually benefiting from those funds. An analysis revealed that African-American residents living in predominantly African-American neighborhoods and CBOs have received fewer benefits from the CDBG program than revealed by the aggregate analysis.

In summary, the mere presence of African-American council members on the CDPC, African Americans living within the CDBG boundaries, or their representation on CBOs' staff or board of directors did not ensure reception of a fair share of CDBG dollars. These efforts seemed more symbolic than meaningful.

On the other hand, the negative impact of race seemed to be more detrimental to African-American neighborhoods and CBOs for several reasons. Some Caucasian CBOs were located in minority areas and served a predominantly African-American clientele. Caucasians dominated the board of directors and professional staff in these agencies. Caucasians were making all the major decisions (contracting work, hiring staff, and purchasing) for the use of CDBG funds in the African-American neighborhoods. Besides making these decisions, they were taking the jobs and money associated with them, thus limiting the recycling of those CDBG dollars into African-American areas. This hindered the development of African-American neighborhoods. Some respondents believed that African-American CBOs were penalized more harshly than Caucasian CBOs. They were more likely to lose their funding or have restrictions placed on them than Caucasian CBOs. Such dual standards resulted in fewer African-American CBOs being available to provide services in African-American neighborhoods. This created major service voids that created other socioeconomic problems. The reduction of African-American CBOs reduced the chances that such agencies would provide professional job opportunities and work experience for many of the African-American residents. The decline of African-American CBOs further removed a valuable link for residents to city government, which provided these funds.

Prominent Caucasian and African-American individuals believed that the use of CDBG funds to replace tax-levy funds for CIPs was very detrimental to the African-American community. If both funding sources had been used, the impact on the African-American community could have been greater. This point could be understood in light of one African-American council member's proud boast, "During my tenure, my aldermanic district has received over $35 million in CDBG funds." Although this person should be proud that her aldermanic district received these CDBG funds, it leads one to ask how much more would have gone to that district if CDBG funds were used to supplement rather than replace tax-levy dollars? The allocation of a large share of CDBG dollars to city agencies meant that African Americans had less input into how those funds were spent. Once municipal agencies received their share of CDBG dollars, there was little, if any, public scrutiny of those funds by the African-American community. These dollars paid for numerous professional positions and provided millions of dollars for the procurement of services and goods beyond the reach of African-American constituents. As city agencies continued to receive a large share of CDBG dollars, African-American neighborhoods and CBOs were further removed from CDBG funding. Finally, African-American neighborhoods and CBOs appeared to be facing a grimmer prospect for CDBG funds. As other minority populations (Asians, Native Americans, Hispanics) grew and matured, they were competing with African-American neighborhoods for CDBG funds. With increased competition from those groups for less CDBG dollars, the amount of CDBG funds going to African-American CBOs and neighborhoods declined.

Chapter 5

CDBG Allocation Patterns

This chapter explores the CDBG distribution patterns under two different mayoral administrations, Maier and Norquist, to determine what role race played in the CDBG allocation patterns. To highlight trends and significant features of CDBG allocation patterns made in each administration, this chapter will focus on, but not be limited to, a comparison of three years under Mayor Maier, 1975, 1980, and 1985, and two years under Mayor Norquist, 1990 and 1995. Data from 1988 to 1997 will be used to illustrate funding trends under Mayor Norquist's administrations. The data from these years clearly indicate that the mayor's office/recommendations were the most important steps in the CDBG funding process. In each funding year, the CDPC accepted a majority of the mayor/CBGA's recommendations. This acceptance rate ranged from a low of 58 percent in 1980 to roughly 67 percent of its CDBG recommendations in 1985, 68.9 percent in 1990, and 87.1 percent in 1995. The common council has been even less reluctant to change the recommendations stemming from the CDPC. During Mayor Maier's years, the common council accepted 66.7 percent in 1980, and 88.6 percent in 1985 of CDPC's recommendations. Although these figures indicate relatively little common council action, compared to the Norquist years, the council was interventionist during Mayor Maier's years. Through 1990 and 1995, the full council changed only one of 259 of CDPC's CDBG recommendations (see Tables 5.1, 5.2, 5.3, and 5.4).

In the crucial first step of the funding process—the mayor/CBGA office's recommendations—African-American CBOs were more likely than Caucasian CBOs to be recommended for no funding. In two years (1985-1986 and 1995), a similar percentage of African-American CBOs and Caucasian CBOs were recommended for no CDBG

TABLE 5.1. CDBG Trace Analysis, 1980 to 1981, Funding Results

Race	NF	R	I	K	S	M	T
Level 1: CBGA/Mayor's Recommendations							
AA	15	10	1	0	2	0	28
C	14	19	1	0	1	1	35
O	4	2	0	0	2	0	8
M	10	0	0	0	0	0	10
T	43	31	2	0	5	1	81
Level 2: CDPC's Recommendations							
AA	4	0	11	1	12	0	28
C	2	1	13	0	19	0	35
O	2	0	0	0	16	0	18
M	0	0	0	0	0	0	0
T	8	1	24	1	47	0	81
Level 3: Council's Recommendations							
AA	2	3	6	0	17	0	28
C	1	1	11	0	22	0	35
O	0	0	3	0	5	0	8
M	0	0	0	0	10	0	10
T	3	4	20	0	54	0	81

Source: CBGA, 1980

NF = No Funds; R = Reduced; I = Increased; K = Kept Open; S = Same; M = Missing; T = Total

funding by the mayor's office/CBGA. However, in both 1980 and 1990, African-American CBOs were much more likely to fall victim to the mayor's/CBGA's cuts. In 1980, 53.6 percent of African-American CBOs' CDBG proposals and only 40 percent of Caucasian CDBG proposals were recommended for no CDBG funding. In 1990, almost half of all African-American CBO proposals (48.8 percent) and less than one-third of Caucasian CBOs' requests (31.0 percent) were recommended for no CDBG funding.

In addition to the matter of CBO proposals being denied, this chapter will also examine the distribution of CDBG dollars in the various

TABLE 5.2. CDBG Trace Analysis, 1985 to 1986, Funding Results

Race	NF	R	I	K	S	M	T
Level 1: CBGA/Mayor's Recommendations							
AA	18	12	0	0	0	0	30
C	34	19	0	0	0	0	53
O	3	1	0	0	0	0	4
M	10	0	0	0	0	0	10
T	65	32	0	0	0	0	97
Level 2: CDPC's Recommendations							
AA	0	3	10	0	17	0	30
C	1	1	16	0	35	0	53
O	0	1	0	0	3	0	4
M	0	0	0	0	10	0	10
T	1	5	26	0	65	0	97
Level 3: Council's Recommendations							
AA	1	0	3	0	26	0	30
C	1	0	6	0	46	0	53
O	0	0	0	0	4	0	4
M	0	0	0	0	10	0	10
T	2	0	9	0	86	0	97

Source: CBGA, 1985

NF = No Funds; R = Reduced; I = Increased; K = Kept Open; S = Same; M = Missing; T = Total

aldermanic or city council districts over time. The central question addressed in this analysis was the degree to which CDBG funds were flowing to majority African-American aldermanic districts. The relevant data to answer this question is contained in Table 5.5. From 1980 to 1990, there were three such aldermanic districts: the first, sixth, and tenth. With the aldermanic redistricting in 1992, the newly created seventeenth aldermanic district became majority African-Amerians. The seventh aldermanic district also became a majority African-American district in 1992 and was represented by an African Ameri-

TABLE 5.3. CDBG Trace Analysis, 1990, Funding Results

Race	NF	R	I	K	S	M	T
Level 1: CBGA/Mayor's Recommendations							
AA	20	19	1	1	0	0	41
C	18	25	4	2	9	0	58
O	5	3	0	0	0	0	8
M	11	1	0	0	0	0	12
T	54	48	5	3	9	0	119
Level 2: CDPC's Recommendations							
AA	0	1	10	4	26	0	41
C	3	1	14	0	40	0	58
O	0	0	2	2	4	0	8
M	0	0	0	0	12	0	12
T	3	2	26	6	82	0	119
Level 3: Council's Recommendations							
AA	0	0	0	0	41	0	41
C	0	1	0	0	57	0	58
O	0	0	0	0	8	0	8
M	0	0	0	0	12	0	12
T	0	1	0	0	118	0	119

Source: CBGA, 1990

NF = No Funds; R = Reduced; I = Increased; K = Kept Open; S = Same; M = Missing; T = Total

can. The total share of CDBG funds received by CBOs in African-American aldermanic districts increased appreciatively from a low of 6.4 percent in 1980 to a peak of 21 percent in 1990. Still, there was a decline in 1995 to 13 percent, a decrease from the previous two time periods.

At first glance, this trend appeared to indicate that Milwaukee's African-American community had increasingly benefited from the CDBG program. Yet it is important to disaggregate these figures and determine if these CDBG dollars flowing to the African-American aldermanic districts were going to Caucasian CBOs or African-

TABLE 5.4. CDBG Trace Analysis, 1995, Funding Results

Race	NF	R	I	K	S	M	T
Level 1: CBGA/Mayor's Recommendations							
AA	9	30	3	1	3	0	46
C	12	43	5	4	7	0	71
O	4	7	1	0	0	0	12
M	10	1	0	0	0	0	11
T	35	81	9	5	10	0	140
Level 2: CDPC's Recommendations							
AA	0	0	4	2	40	0	46
C	0	2	7	2	60	0	71
O	0	1	0	0	11	0	12
M	0	0	0	0	11	0	11
T	0	3	11	4	122	0	140
Level 3: Council's Recommendations							
AA	0	0	0	0	46	0	46
C	0	0	0	0	71	0	71
O	0	0	0	0	12	0	12
M	0	0	0	0	11	0	11
T	0	0	0	0	140	0	140

Source: CBGA, 1995b

NF = No Funds; R = Reduced; I = Increased; K = Kept Open; S = Same; M = Missing; T = Total

American CBOs. The data necessary to examine this trend are contained in Table 5.6. African-American CBOs received roughly 70 percent of CDBG funds in majority African-American aldermanic districts in 1980 and 1990, peaking at 81.9 percent in 1985. By 1995, African-American CBOs received just a little more than half (57.8 percent) of CDBG dollars allocated in what were now five majority African-American aldermanic districts. This pattern provided some support to the views of African-American public officials who offered anecdotal evidence about the changing nature of CBOs within

TABLE 5.5. CDBG Funds to African-American Aldermanic Districts, 1980 to 1995 (per $1,000)

Year	CDBG to AA Districts	Total CDBG
1980	1,450	22,795
1985	2,838	17,684
1990	3,253	15,487
1995	2,880	22,000

Source: CBGA (various years)

TABLE 5.6. CDBG by Race to African-American Aldermanic Districts, 1980 to 1995 (per $1,000)

	CBO's Race			
Year	AA	C	O	T
1980	975	421	53	1,449
1985	2,325	512	0	2,837
1990	2,292	961	0	3,253
1995	2,880	2,075	30	4,985

Source: CBGA (various years)

AA = African American; C = Caucasians; O = Others; T = Total

the city's African-American community. It is also a caution for researchers to look beyond aggregate numbers when studying CDBG distribution patterns in aldermanic districts.

Examining the distribution of CDBG funds by aldermanic districts without looking at the CBOs funded in those areas may be misleading for several reasons. It may not reveal which CBOs, in terms of racial composition of directors and staff, were receiving CDBG funds in those aldermanic districts. Because an aldermanic district was considered majority African-American did not mean that CDBG funds were going to African-American CBOs in those areas. African Americans might not have made decisions related to the jobs associated with operating those CBOs. The results in Tables 5.7, 5.8, 5.9, and

TABLE 5.7. CDBG Dollars by Race of CBO to Aldermanic Districts, 1980 to 1981 (per $1,000)

Districts	AA	C	O	T
01*	157	0	0	157
02	0	0	0	0
03	0	0	0	0
04	384	686	0	1,070
05	0	0	0	0
06*	796	322	53	1,171
07	103	418	0	521
08	0	424	0	424
09	0	599	0	599
10	22	99	0	121
11	0	0	0	0
12	0	578	832	1,410
13	0	0	0	0
14	0	0	0	0
15	0	270	0	270
16	0	0	0	0
17	0	0	0	0
99**	0	0	0	0
T	1,462	3,396	885	5,743

Source: CBGA, 1980
AA = African American; C = Caucasians; O = Others; T = Total
*AA Districts
**Missing

5.10 showed that African-American CBOs did not receive a major share of CDBG funds awarded to majority Caucasian aldermanic districts. African-American CBOs only received CDBG funds in one Caucasian aldermanic district, district four. Whereas Caucasian CBOs were a significant provider of services in African-American aldermanic districts, African-American CBOs were not major service providers in Caucasian aldermanic districts.

TABLE 5.8. CDBG Dollars by Race of CBO to Aldermanic Districts, 1985 to 1986 (per $1,000)

Districts	AA	C	O	T
01*	510	87	0	597
02	0	0	0	0
03	0	0	120	120
04	506	1,070	0	1,576
05	0	0	0	0
06*	1,115	375	0	1,490
07	0	481	0	481
08	0	600	0	600
09	0	0	0	0
10*	700	50	0	750
11	0	0	0	0
12	0	524	0	524
13	0	0	0	0
14	0	0	0	0
15	0	0	0	0
16	179	0	0	179
17	0	0	0	0
99**	0	0	0	0
T	3,010	3,187	120	6,317

Source: CBGA, 1985
AA = African American; C = Caucasians; O = Others; T = Total
*AA Districts
**Missing

The role of race in the distribution of CDBG funds in Milwaukee changed over the years. During Mayor Maier's administrations, race played the biggest role relative to the use of CDBG funds for CIPs. Some African-American and Caucasian council members believed that Mayor Maier's administrations were biased against the African-American neighborhoods because CDBG funds were used to supplant tax-levy dollars for CIPs. The decision to use CDBG funds for

TABLE 5.9. CDBG Dollars by Race of CBO to Aldermanic Districts, 1990 (Per $1,000)

Districts	AA	C	O	T
01*	397	150	0	547
02	0	52	0	52
03	0	0	0	0
04	610	2,061	0	2,671
05	0	0	0	0
06*	1,012	764	0	1,777
07	389	551	0	940
08	0	592	0	592
09	0	0	0	0
10*	882	47	0	929
11	0	0	0	0
12	0	1,304	180	1,484
13	0	0	0	0
14	0	0	0	0
15	0	0	0	0
16	70	70	0	140
17	0	0	0	0
99**	0	21	0	21
T	3,360	5612	180	9,153

Source: CBGA, 1990
AA = African American; C = Caucasians; O = Others; T = Total
*AA Districts
**Missing

CIPs meant that there was a shrinking allotment of CDBG funds allocated to African-American neighborhoods. CDBG allocations examined and presented in the tables in this chapter provide statistical support to this perspective.

When the CDBG allocation patterns were further analyzed by council district allocations, two significant patterns emerged. Under Mayor Maier's administrations a larger percentage of CDBG funds were allocated for CIP purposes than under Mayor Norquist's admin-

TABLE 5.10. CDBG Dollars by Race of CBO to Aldermanic Districts, 1995 (per $1,000)

Districts	AA	C	O	T
01*	187	346	0	533
02	0	0	0	0
03	0	889	0	899
04	75	2,809	195	3,079
05	0	0	0	0
06*	956	0	0	956
07*	712	50	0	762
08	0	627	0	627
09	0	0	0	0
10*	524	574	0	1,098
11	0	0	0	0
12	0	1,155	658	1,813
13	0	0	0	0
14	0	50	0	50
15	0	0	0	0
16	0	0	0	0
17*	500	1,105	30	635
99**	0	0	0	0
T	2,954	7,605	883	11,442

Source: CBGA, 1995a
AA = African American; C = Caucasians; O = Others; T = Total
*AA Districts
** Missing

istrations. Another pattern showed more CDBG dollars went for CIPs in African-American communities than Caucasian neighborhoods under Mayor Maier (see Table 5.11). Although Mayor Maier spent from a low of $3.2 million of CDBG dollars for CIPs in 1985 to a high of $10.1 million in 1980, Mayor Norquist did not finance any CIPs with CDBG funds in either 1990 or 1995. The results in Table 5.11 reveal that the use of CDBG funds for CIPs changed over time

TABLE 5.11. CDBG for CIPs in African-American Aldermanic Districts, 1975 to 1995 (per $1,000)

Year	Total CDBG	CDBG for CIP	CDBG for CIP in AA
1975	13,383	7,823	1,487
1980	22,754	10,107	1,223
1985	17,684	3,218	1,868
1990	15,328	0	0
1995	22,000	0	0

Source: CBGA (various years)
AA = African American Districts

by aldermanic districts. In 1975 and 1980, Mayor Maier's administrations distributed these capital improvement projects in a rough proportional to the city's racial makeup. In 1985 almost 58 percent of CDBG-funded CIPs were located in African-American aldermanic districts. In the end, by choosing to use CDBG allotments to fund so many CIPs in African-American neighborhoods, Mayor Maier's administrations in essence reduced the share of CDBG funds available to African-American CBOs operating in African-American neighborhoods.

Although the use of CDBG funds for capital improvement projects was a point of contention during Mayor Maier's administrations, the defunding and reduction of CDBG dollars to African-American CBOs was controversial in the African-American community during Mayor Norquist's administrations from 1988 to 1997. Under Mayor Norquist, African-American CBOs experienced major cuts in the three largest funding areas (housing, economic development, and public services).

African-American CBOs involved in housing production suffered drastically during Mayor Norquist's administrations. Housing production involved the acquisition and renovation of primarily foreclosed, boarded, or substandard housing units. Once these properties were completed, they were sold to low- and moderate-income fami-

TABLE 5.12. CDBG Housing Production (per $1,000)

	CBO's Race			
Year	AA	C	O	T
1988	320	1,219	0	1,539
1989	441	1,641	0	2,082
1990	386	1,360	70	1,816
1991	186	1,394	56	1,636
1992	679	1,733	80	2,492
1993	180	1,083	0	1,263
1994	226	1,243	0	1,469
1995	229	1,629	90	1,948
1996	245	1,996	100	2,341
1997	0	1,626	0	1,620
T	2,892	14,924	396	18,212

Source: CBGA (various years)
AA = African Americans; C = Caucasians; O = Others; T = Total

lies per HUD's requirements. This program was designed to encourage neighborhood stability and ensure the availability of affordable housing. Table 5.12 showed the following patterns:

1. Between 1988 and 1997, African-American housing production CBOs received an annual average of 15.9 percent of the CDBG funds awarded for this category.
2. The percentage of CDBG dollars awarded to African-American housing production CBOs declined from 20.8 percent in 1988 to 0 percent in 1997.
3. The percentage of CDBG funds allocated to African-American housing production CBOs declined steadily each year after 1990, with one exception that occurred in 1992, when they received a high of 27.1 percent of CDBG funds.
4. Prior to 1997, Milwaukee United for Better Housing (MUFBH) was the only African-American housing production CBO that had been funded each year during the Norquist's years.

5. In 1997, MUFBH was provided $1 in CDBG funds to allow it to carryover unspent 1996 CDBG funds. Its request for carryover funding was later denied, resulting in this program being defunded.

6. By 1997 all African-American housing production CBOs had been defunded and closed.

In addition to a decline in funds for housing production activities, African-American CBOs suffered significant cuts in the housing production–others category. This category focused on housing projects that addressed an urgent community need or leveraged significant resources for neighborhood revitalization efforts. See Table 5.13. Those trends were as follows:

1. The percentage of CDBG dollars for housing production–others awarded to African-American CBOs between 1993 and 1997 was 54.0 percent.

2. One project (New Covenant) accounted for the majority of the CDBG funds for African-American housing production–others CBOs in 1995 and 1996.

3. The percentage of CDBG funds going to African-American housing production–others decreased from a high of 68.3 percent in 1995 to 0 percent in 1997.

4. By 1997, no African-American CBO involved in housing production–others received new CDBG dollars during the regular CDBG funding cycle.

TABLE 5.13. CDBG Housing Production–Others (per $1,000)

	CBO's Race			
Year	AA	C	O	T
1993	150	0	0	150
1994	100	535	50	685
1995	606	281	0	887
1996	700	350	0	1,050
1997	0	75	0	75
T	1,556	1,241	50	2,847

Source: CBGA (various years)
AA = African Americans; C = Caucasians; O = Others, T = Total

TABLE 5.14. CDBG Housing NIPs (per $1,000)

	CBO's Race			
Year	AA	C	O	T
1988	1,822	1,675	0	3,497
1989	1,551	1,777	0	3,328
1990	1,771	2,027	0	3,798
1991	1,660	1,898	0	3,559
1992	1,788	1,917	0	3,706
1993	1,177	1,563	0	2,741
1994	1,336	1,369	0	2,705
1995	1,447	1,767	0	3,215
1996	2,140	3,144	0	5,284
1997	935	2,556	0	3,491
T	15,629	19,696	0	35,326

Source: CBGA, 1996a
AA = African Americans; C = Caucasians; O = Others; T = Total

African-American CBOs receiving funds for housing rehabilitation projects saw a significant decrease in their funding during Mayor Norquist's administrations. These projects were known as neighborhood improvement projects (NIPs). These CBOs provided home repairs to eligible homeowners up to a prescribed cost cap for the correction of housing code violations. CBOs funded in this area provided housing security installation, accessibility, or maintenance support for homeowners. The data in Table 5.14 indicate the following trend:

1. African-American housing CBOs involved in housing rehabilitation received 44.2 percent of the total funds awarded to CBOs.
2. The percentage of CDBG funds to African-American CBOs decreased by almost half for this category, from a high of 52.1 percent in 1988 to 26.8 percent in 1997.
3. The number of African-American CBOs involved in housing rehabilitation decreased from seven in 1988 to two in 1997.
4. Only two African-American CBOs (OIC and Harambee) involved in housing rehabilitation received CDBG funding each year of this study.

5. In 1997, only two African-American CBOs were awarded new CDBG dollars (OIC and Harambee). Even then, they received reductions of $21,000 and $375,000, respectively, from their previous year's CDBG allocation.
6. In 1997, Mayor Norquist vetoed Social Development Commission (SDCs) CDBG funds of $205,000 for its Crime Prevention for Senior Citizens Housing Program, the first veto in the history of the city's CDBG program. SDC had met all of its program performance goals, and it did not have any fiscal problems with them.

These findings had serious implications for the city's African-American community. As African-American housing CBOs were defunded, African-American employees of these CBOs lost their jobs. See Table 5.15. This table shows that African-American CBOs were clearly more likely to hire African Americans. Based on the last program year of available data (1994 to 1995), 83.9 percent of the employees of African-American CBOs were African Americans. In contrast, African Americans constituted 41 percent of employees in Caucasian housing CBOs. With the defunding of the Commandos Incorporation, MUFBH, and O. C. White Soul Club, twenty-nine employees, including twenty-eight African Americans, lost their jobs. With the defunding of the Commandos, the Milwaukee Christian Center (MCC), a Caucasian CBO, was awarded $160,000 in 1997 to construct handicap-accessible ramps, a task previously performed by the Commandos. This illustrates the loss in jobs for African-Ameri-

TABLE 5.15. CBOs' CDBG-Funded Positions, 1996

CBOs'race	Employees' Race			
	AA	**C**	**O**	**T**
AA	89	20	5	114
C	227	234	72	533
O	2	7	23	32
T	318	261	100	679

Source: CBGA, 1996a
AA = African Americans; C = Caucasians; O = Others; T = Total

can employees when African-American housing CBOs lost their funding and Caucasian CBOs replaced them.

Similarly, the defunding of African-American housing CBOs obviously impacted their ability to subcontract work to other groups or businesses. Table 5.16 shows the reduction of subcontracting activities by African-American contractors after the defunding of some African-American CBOs:

1. In 1995 to 1996, African-American contractors were awarded $293,150 or 8.3 percent of the total subcontracting dollars that year. Caucasian contractors were awarded $3.2 million or 91.6 percent of the $3,508,904 in housing subcontracting activities.
2. In 1996 to 1997 African-American contractors accounted for only $1,681 or less than 1 percent of the $1.9 million in housing subcontracting dollars awarded that year. Caucasian contractors accounted for $1,989,733 or 99.9 percent of all subcontracting dollars awarded that year.
3. Between 1995 and 1996, African-American contractors' subcontracting activities decreased from $293,150 to $1,681 in 1996 to 1997, a loss of $291,469, or −99.9 percent.
4. Caucasian contractors' subcontracting funding decreased from $3,215,754 in 1995 to 1996 to $1,988,052 in 1996 to 1997, a loss of $1,227,702, or −38.1 percent.

In addition, the quality of housing in the African-American community was left to decline when these African-American housing CBOs were defunded. As one executive director of an African-American housing CBO stated in 1996,

> those properties [vacant and boarded-up houses] will remain vacant and a blight on the community instead of being a stabilizing force in the community. The longer those properties are allowed to sit, the more expensive it becomes to rehabilitate them because of vandalism, deterioration; thereby reducing the availability of affordable and safe housing for the community.

Similarly, these vacant properties become potential sites for criminal activities (drug dealing, arson). These deteriorated and vacant houses

TABLE 5.16. CDBG CBOs' Subcontracting Dollars to Contractors (per $1,000)

Contractors'	1995-1996	1996-1997	Change
AA	293	1	292
C	3,215	1,998	1,217
T	3,508	1,999	1,509

Source: CBGA (various years)
AA = African Americans; C = Caucasians; T = Total

contributed to declining property values in the area. Finally, these vacant and boarded-up houses resulted in lost tax revenue because they were not on the city's tax roll.

African-American CBOs also suffered a decreased share of CDBG funds for economic development projects. This category provided CDBG funds for a variety of activities: commercial or industrial improvements, job creation, loans and grants for small business development, and technical assistance (see Table 5.17). African-American CBOs' share of CDBG funding for economic development projects were subject to the following trends:

1. Between 1988 and 1997, African-American CBOs received an annual average 29.3 percent of CDBG funds for economic development activities.
2. CDBG funds for African-American CBOs for economic development projects decreased from a high of 46.8 percent in 1988 to 18 percent in 1997.
3. With the exception of 1992, the percentage of CDBG funds awarded to African-American CBOs for economic development activities decreased in each year of this study.
4. In 1997, African-American CBOs received their lowest percentage of CDBG dollars for economic development activities, 18 percent.
5. Only one African-American agency, Milwaukee Urban League, received CDBG funds every year of this study for economic development activities.
6. Since 1994, fewer than three African-American CBOs have been funded in a given year for economic development activities.

TABLE 5.17. CDBG Economic Development Dollars Awarded to CBOs (per $1,000)

Year	CBOs' Race			
	AA	**C**	**O**	**T**
1988	305	266	80	651
1989	380	498	60	938
1990	365	610	0	975
1991	515	706	85	1,306
1992	160	0	80	240
1993	393	612	80	1,085
1994	245	676	105	1,026
1995	325	930	115	1,370
1996	345	676	130	1,151
1997	420	1,745	130	2,295
T	3,453	6,719	865	11,037

Source: CBGA (various years)
AA = African Americans; C = Caucasians; O = Others; T = Total

This decline of African-American CBOs' share of CDBG-funded economic development projects had negative impacts. One impact was that it meant less CDBG funds were available for job training and placement, business loans, technical assistance, and other activities in African-American neighborhoods. These were vital activities needed in the city's African-American community in light of its socioeconomic conditions. It further reduced the potential for businesses relocating or remaining in the area, which could have contributed to both the tax base and the community's stability.

Besides the reduction of CDBG funds for housing and economic development activities, African-American CBOs' share of CDBG dollars for public service projects decreased under Mayor Norquist's administrations. This category includes CDBG funding for numerous programs: community organizing, housing and tenant advocacy, crime prevention, home-owner counseling, youth and recreational activities, elderly assistance, shelters, and so forth. See Table 5.18 for the following trends.

1. Between 1988 and 1997, African-American CBOs received 30.8 percent of all CDBG funds allocated for public service projects.
2. The percentage of CDBG funds for public service projects awarded to African-American CBOs decreased from a high of 37.6 percent in 1989 to 26.3 percent in 1995.
3. Since 1989, the percentage of CDBG funds for public service activities allocated to African-American CBOs have decreased each year.
4. Only two African-American CBOs (SDC-Family Crisis and DOLL) received CDBG funds for public service projects in each year of the study.
5. In 1997, two of the most successful African-American public service programs (SDC's Youth Diversion Program and SDC's Housing Social Services Program) were defunded, despite meeting their performance goals.

In conclusion, the city's African-American community witnessed a significant decrease in CDBG funds, when they were needed the

TABLE 5.18. CDBG Public Service Dollars Awarded to CBOs (per $1,000)

Year	CBOs' Race			
	AA	C	O	T
1988	583	1,092	25	1,700
1989	844	1,374	25	2,243
1990	748	1,223	20	1,991
1991	643	1,282	18	1,943
1992	670	1,559	25	2,254
1993	751	1,506	25	2,282
1994	1,039	2,025	88	3,152
1995	897	2,345	98	3,340
1996	1,115	2,905	114	4,134
1997	1,091	2,915	134	4,140
T	8,381	18,226	572	27,179

Source: CBGA (various years)
AA = African Americans; C = Caucasians; O = Others; T = Total

most. Although some CDBG funds were being allocated to African-American aldermanic districts, African-American CBOs were not getting the bulk of them. Which CBO gets funding is important, as African-American CBOs were twice as likely as Caucasian CBOs to hire African Americans with CDBG funds. On top of depleting valuable jobs and work experience for residents of African-American neighborhoods, the CDBG allocation pattern in Milwaukee revealed that it was increasingly likely that CDBG monies were contributing to the loss of subcontracting and business opportunities within African-American communities. These CDBG reductions occurred across the three largest categories (housing, economic development, and public services). Even though the African-American community's depressing socioeconomic conditions and blight have contributed heavily to the city's poverty rate, which were major factors in the city receiving CDBG funds, the African-American community was benefiting less from the CDBG program.

Chapter 6

The Unequal and Ugly Effect of Race
in the Allocation of CDBG Funds

Although CDBG allocation patterns showed that race did have an impact in funding, the interviews with participants and reviews of government files offered additional evidence of bias against African Americans. The distribution of power and personnel in Milwaukee during this study period resulted in these biases working against African-American CBOs. These biases were manifested in unfair and racist performance evaluation of African-American CBOs, and the termination of cash advances. Specifically, numerous instances occurred in which Caucasian CBOs benefited and African-American CBOs were penalized in the CDBG funding process due to these pre-existing biases.

Prior to April 1996 when the CDPC hired its staff to review CDBG proposals, make funding recommendations, and conduct CDBG policy analysis, the review of all CDBG proposals was CBGA's sole responsibility. The CBGA would then make funding recommendations, in consultation with the mayor's office, before making them public. There were several flaws with this evaluation process. One problem was that the CDPC members were totally dependent on the CBGA staff for an objective analysis of CDBG proposals and CDBG policy issues. A second problem was that the information provided by the CBGA was sometimes misleading, incomplete, and biased. Some African-American CBOs, which met or exceeded all of their CDBG performance goals, were denied funding because CBGA's write-ups indicated that those programs had "poor performance."

Two examples illustrate this point. The Social Development Commission (SDC), the largest African-American CBO faced such a fate. SDC's youth diversion program met or exceeded all its performance goals in 1995 and 1996 and had received both local and national recognition for its accomplishments. It was denied 1996 closeout funds and new CDBG funding in 1997 by the CBGA/mayor's office because of its alleged poor performance, which was not the case. The common council's staff prepared a report on the SDC's performance using CBGA's data, which showed that the SDC had the city's best performing CDBG program. Its four CDBG-funded programs (Crime Prevention for Senior Citizens, Family Crisis Center, Housing Social Services, and Youth Diversion) met or exceeded a combined fifteen of seventeen (88 percent) of their goals in 1995. Sometimes they exceeded program goals by more than 1,000 percent. By June 1996, all four of its CDBG-funded programs had already met or were on schedule to meet their program goals for 1996 (Gordon, personal communication, 1996). Yet the mayor's office/CBGA recommended no funding for three of those programs: Youth Diversion, Crime Prevention for Senior Citizens, and Housing Social Services.

The CDPC recommended $310,000 for the SDC's programs (Crime Prevention, Fighting Back Initiative, etc.). The CDPC "chose" not to recommend funding for the Youth Diversion Program because the mayor had indicated he was going to veto its funding. In an attempt to provide an "olive branch" to the mayor to prevent him from vetoing funding for the other funded programs, the CDPC did not provide funding for it. This attempted compromise would later fail after the common council supported those CDPC recommendations. The mayor later vetoed funding for three SDC Programs (Housing Social Services, Crime Prevention for Seniors, Fighting Back Initiative) because of its alleged management problems with non-CDBG-related programs. The council sustained his veto. The CDPC was not able to override the mayor's veto. A portion of the SDC's funding was later conditionally restored.

The CDPC and common council were aware that the the SDC's CDBG-funded programs had met or exceeded all their performance goals. Some council members expressed opposition to SDC programs based on feedback from voters in their districts, who opposed this agency's funding. Even the mayor's office and the CBGA could not dispute the common council staff's analysis that showed SDC had some of the best performing CDBG-funded programs. Instead, the CBGA director stated that although there "were some problems" at the programs and some "duplication of services" with other agencies, "contract objectives were being met" (Norman, 1996c, p. B4).

Besides the lack of performance problems, the SDC's CDBG-funded programs did not have any fiscal or management problems. The SDC's previous management staff had some questionable credentials and there were some concerns with a few air conditioners not being delivered to elderly residents, and although these concerns were legitimate concerns and received a great deal of attention from the local media, these troubles were not associated with its CDBG-funded projects. Still, the SDC was denied some funds based on those concerns. Once the SDC's funding was denied, elected representatives from the City of Milwaukee, Milwaukee County, and other interested parties forced the SDC to restructure.

The Carpenter's Incorporated, another African-American housing CBO, met all of its performance goals in 1996 but was denied new funding and a carryover request because of alleged "poor performance" and concerns about it not submitting some CDBG cost reports which showed the CBO's CDBG expenditures. In testimony before the CDPC, the CBO's executive director stated that the CBGA withheld the CBO's actual performance data. She stated that the CBGA, prior to the CDPC's review of that agency's proposal, had been provided accurate and updated information which showed that the group met its performance goals. The agency had completed twenty-nine housing units, although it was only contracted to complete twenty-five. Accurate performance information on this group was not provided until the CBGA's recommendation for this group had been made and its executive director came to the CDPC meeting with this data. The CBO's executive director called Michael Bonds to inform him of this matter after the CBGA had already provided the CDPC with the inaccurate performance data. This group was not awarded any CDBG funds during the regular CDBG funding cycle in fall 1996, but it would later be awarded $370,000 in CDBG reprogramming dollars in June 1997, eight months later. The Carpenter's Incorporated, however, would later be defunded in 1998 for alleged breach of contract (not filing some legal papers with Milwaukee County, which costs less than $30 per property).

In summary, these two cases offer some evidence that African-American CBOs, which had met or exceeded their goals, were described in an inaccurate and negative light by the CBGA in its review of CDBG proposals and write-ups provided to the CDPC members. Without its own staff to provide an independent analysis of CDBG proposals and review performance data, the CDPC was left to depend on the information of the CBGA, which did not always provide complete and accurate information. As one African-American CDBG monitor stated in 1996, "this practice has been going on for years and African-American groups have been getting screwed as a result of it." Similarly, in 1996, one Hispanic CDBG monitor stated, "We are 'told' to change our analysis of groups to portray them in a particular way."

The practice of terminating cash advances to CBOs was used in a biased way against African-American CBOs. Several African-American CBOs and several Caucasian CBOs encountered program performance or financial problems, but they were treated differently. Through the comptroller's office, the CDBG program offered all CDBG-funded CBOs a cash advance of their CDBG funds, which is the equivalent of forty-five days of CDBG funds that CBOs use as "operating capital" until other funds become available. CBOs could obtain a cash advance at any point during the CDBG funding year. For many CBOs, especially African-American CBOs that had limited or no other funding sources, the use of the cash advance enabled them to operate until other monies become available since CDBG funds were provided on a reimbursable basis. Cash advance payments were deducted from future CBO's monthly CDBG payments.

The city government's standard practice was to pull the cash advance from any CBO that had tax problems, a lien or judgment against it, or other fiscal problems. With good reason, the city regulators believed that a CBO facing such difficulties could lose the cash advance as a result of a dispute with a creditor. Although this policy was initiated as a safeguard to make sure that CDBG funds were spent on intended purposes, public officials applied this standard in an inconsistent and biased manner, using it as a tool to withhold monies from African-American CBOs.

The practice of terminating the cash advances, in some instances, operated to the disadvantage of African-American CBOs, which were held to higher performance and administrative standards than were Caucasian CBOs. Several African-American CBOs involved in housing-related activities (Commandos, O. C. White Soul Club, MUFBH) had their cash advance terminated, or had their CDBG contracts terminated when it was revealed that they had fiscal problems, management problems, or legal problems.

The Commandos Incorporation, an African-American housing CBO involved in the construction of handicap-accessible ramps, had its cash advance pulled in 1995 when its problems were revealed. According to the 1996 CDBG *Briefing Book,* "the project is facing financial problems that jeopardize its viability. The Wisconsin Department of Revenue is owed about $11,000 in withholding taxes and the comptroller has pulled the program's $30,000 cash advance" (CBGA, 1996a, p. 193.) The Commandos Incorporation reported that due to errors by its former accountant (billing on the net pay instead of the gross pay), it owed $14,000 in federal taxes and $2,700 in state taxes. Those errors were corrected, when they were identified, and all but $1,947 in back taxes were paid (Clark, personal communication, 1996; Wade, personal communication, 1996). The Commandos' cash advance was pulled immediately.

When the Commando's cash advance was pulled, it was one of the better performing CDBG-funded housing programs, as listed in Table 6.1. In 1991, the Commandos completed thirty-one of thirty-two planned handicapped ramps. In 1992, the Commandos completed 100 percent of planned ramps. The CBGA noted,

> In each of the last four years, the program has met its production goal. In 1993, the agency completed 24 of 24 units. In 1994, for example, it completed 74 bi-approved ramps, slightly surpassing its ramp production goal of 73. As of June 1996, it had completed 21 ramps (24 planned) which is near production capacity. (CBGA, 1996a, p. 193)

TABLE 6.1. Commando's Housing Performance Data, 1991 to 1995, Housing Unit Performance

Year	Completed	Proposed	% of Proposed
1991	31	32	96.9
1992	32	32	100.0
1993	24	24	100.0
1994	74	73	101.0
1995	49	60	81.7

Source: CBGA, 1996a

The Commandos Incorporation would eventually complete twenty-four of twenty-four units proposed that year. The only year the Commandos did not reach its production goals during this five-year period was in 1995, the year its cash advance was taken. In 1995, the Commandos completed forty-nine of sixty (82 percent) proposed units without a cash advance.

The Commandos Incorporation would later have its CDBG funds eliminated in 1996 for 1997, once it was revealed that the CBGA had received a tax levy notice in excess of $189,000 against the agency for not withholding and paying appropriate taxes. The 1997 *Briefing Book* also noted other problems (poor filing system, accounting and administrative concerns, questions regarding the submittal of cost reports, missing invoices, missing cancelled checks) with the agency. Rather than assist this successfully performing agency, this CBO was defunded and forced to close (CBGA, 1993-1997). Its work for constructing handicap-accessible ramps was later awarded to a Caucasian agency, Milwaukee Christian Center, for $160,000 via two contracts.

Milwaukee United for Better Housing (MUFBH), another African-American housing CBO, lost its cash advance when it encountered problems in 1993. Conflicting views were provided about the specific nature of this agency's problems. On the one hand, the 1993 CDBG *Briefing Book* noted that cost claims were made for items not budgeted and there were some duplicated claims, which led to the reimbursement for two properties totaling $39,000. The city paid another $7,675 in duplicated costs. MUFBH eventually paid the city $15,000 and owed it $31,675 when the cash advance was pulled. An on-site audit by the comptroller's office in 1996 found problems with the agency's accounting system. Likewise, the agency's general ledger had not been posted since May 1995. Documentation was missing for two checks totaling $1,511. Finally, the agency submitted $14,260 in cost reports from the city, but the checks had not been released to the vendors, which was contrary to the city's CBGA policies. Those checks were later replaced and released to the vendors (CBGA, 1993-1997).

On the other hand, the agency's executive director provided a different view of those events. He indicated MUFBH had its cash advance terminated for minor fiscal problems. In 1991, the agency had not turned in receipts to the city showing expenditures of $150,000 in

CDBG funds because of a bad record-keeping system. Those receipts for supplies related to the repair of housing units were eventually located and provided to the city in 1992. Not only did the agency provide the city with those receipts, but it also claimed it found an additional $50,000 worth of receipts for which it was entitled to reimbursement from the city. The agency's executive director indicated that the comptroller's office later acknowledged that the agency provided the receipts, and it was entitled to $50,000 in reimbursement. This agency never had its cash advance restored, nor was it given the $50,000. MUFBH's performance declined significantly once it lost its cash advance in 1991. See Table 6.2.

In October 1995, O. C. White Soul Club had its CDBG NIP contract for housing rehabilitation terminated, effective in 1996, for performance purposes (Norman, 1995). O. C. White Soul Club had some administrative and program performance problems. The CBGA *Briefing Books* for the period 1993 to 1996 indicated that the agency had the following problems: cash advances were consistently out of balance; there were inadequate accounting procedures and problems with its general ledger; tax payment withholdings were deposited late; and several thousand dollars of CDBG funds were used for ineligible expenses. The agency had missing checks and late bills, and its housing rehabilitation costs had been higher than average. These problems contributed to the agency's demise as it lost its cash advance. "The decision by the Comptroller's Office to rescind the Cash Advance was pursuant to an IRS judgment of $28,000+ for the Soul

TABLE 6.2. MUFBH's Housing Performance Data, 1989 to 1995, Housing Unit Performance

Year	Completed	Proposed	% Completed
1989	7	9	77.8
1990	6	19	31.6
1991	12	15	80.0
1992	1	15	6.7
1993	5	20	25.0
1994	6	20	30.0
1995	1	22	4.0

Source: CBGA (various years)

Club's failure to pay employee withholding taxes from March through December, 1994" (CBGA, 1996a, p. 18).

The agency had some performance problems. Between 1991 and 1993, it was contracted to complete 135 housing units, but completed only 67 percent. In 1993, the agency received a contract for 42.5 housing units, but finished only 25.5 (60 percent). Between 1990 and 1992, it had completed 75 percent (30 of 40), 69 percent (30.5 of 44), and 72 percent (35 of 48.5) of its projected goals.

The O. C. White Soul Club already had its cash advance pulled because of these problems, but it was later reinstated in 1994. The CDPC had provided the agency with an additional $35,000 to hire an accountant to assist with the agency's financial records and provided it $30,000 for 1995 to balance its books (CBGA, 1993-1997). The next year the agency made some program improvements by meeting its 1994 housing production goal of thirty-two units as shown in Table 6.3. Despite making some progress between 1994 and 1995, O. C. White Soul Club lost its cash advance and its CDBG funds in 1996, and it was forced to close (CBGA, 1993-1997).

Although O. C. White Soul Club and other African-American CBOs had some notable problems, when Caucasian CBOs had similar or worse problems, their cash advances and CDBG contracts were not terminated. Three Caucasian CBOs stood out during this study period: Westside Conservation Corporation (WCC); East Side Housing Action Committee, (ESHAC); and the Northwest Side Community Development Corporation (NWSCDC).

WCC, a Caucasian CBO, had numerous fiscal and management problems. Its housing rehabilitation cost $11,000 more per unit than

TABLE 6.3. O. C. White Soul Club's NIP Performance Data, 1990 to 1994, Housing Unit Performance

Year	Completed	Proposed	% of Completed
1990	30	40	75.0
1991	30.5	44	69.3
1992	35	48.5	72.2
1993	25	42.5	58.8
1994	32	32	100.0

Source: CBGA (various years)

expected. Instead of spending $22,000 per unit on a house, WCC spent at least $33,000 per housing unit. In 1994, WCC spent an average of $31,499 per unit; in 1995, this amount rose to $35,640. WCC reported greater than expected costs in buying and maintaining properties, improper estimation of project costs, and city auditors found deficient systems for monitoring contractor invoices. Several firms were awarded court judgments against the agency or had filed liens against its assets (Schuldt, 1997a).

The comptroller's office raised concerns about this CBO's fiscal practices as early as 1992 when it constantly questioned if its CDBG funds were being used appropriately. WCC accumulated more than $200,000 in building code forfeitures and delinquent property tax bills during this period while still receiving new CDBG funds (Schuldt, 1997c).

The comptroller's office listed major concerns about this project in the 1997 CBGA *Briefing Book.* Those concerns included payment of $28,000 in Home Ownership Made Easy (HOME) funds and $11,000 in CDBG funds for work that was undocumented; $11,500 of the $28,000 was related to voided checks, but no replacement checks were issued. Another $16,300 was claimed for work completed on two different properties ($32,600 total), but the work was done on only one property. Included was $2,932 more than the actual check of $29,662 for this claim. Some cost claims were not properly authorized. The agency did not submit a detailed schedule of cash balances for each funding source, and WCC consistently claimed ineligible costs relating to sales taxes or discounts. Its housing program's costs exceeded the $7,000 expected for administrative expenses and $15,000 for direct rehabilitation subsidies. Although the average cost per unit was projected to be $10,000, WCC's costs exceeded $25,000. WCC had six separate cash advances, five of which were not balanced during the comptroller's office site visit. Several months later four of the six remained out of balance (CBGA, 1993-1997).

Besides its fiscal problems, this CBO had some serious program performance problems. The agency failed to meet its housing rehabilitation goals in each year from 1991 through 1996. From 1993 through 1995, it was contracted to complete 145 housing units, but completed only eighty housing units or 55 percent (Schuldt, 1997a). It did not meet its housing rehabilitation goals for three straight years (1993 to 1995) and it was not in a position to meet them in 1996

(Dries, 1996). WCC received numerous complaints of poor work-manship from the owners of the properties it repaired (Schuldt, 1997b; Schuldt, 1997d). WCC received complaints from residents who wanted the group out of its neighborhood for failing to complete the rehabilitation of properties the group bought from a slumlord (Nichols, 1995b).

In 1992, 1993, and 1994, the agency did not meet its performance goals, as shown in Table 6.4. Yet there were some contradictions in the CBGA's reporting of this agency's program performance. The data in Table 6.4 indicate that the project completed twenty-three of forty-five units in 1994. Yet the 1995 CDBG *Briefing Book* indicated that the agency was not on schedule to meet its 1994 goals. It had completed only nine of eighteen units through June 1994. Though auditors sustained these findings, the city described WCC as having met 100 percent of its goals in 1994. Similarly, CBGA prepared a report that showed that in 1994, the agency completed only twenty-three of forty-five (51 percent) of its goals (CBGA, 1996b). The 1996 CBGA *Briefing Book* indicated, "The project is experiencing some difficulty in 1995 (CBGA, 1996a, p. 246)." The CBO's current inventory of projects was purchased several years ago, and it continued to deteriorate. The project exhausted its allocation of housing production funds on its first twenty housing units because of the high cost of property tax and maintenance. Finally, the former CBGA director indicated, "the nonprofit housing agency also failed to meet its rehabilitation goals from 1991 through 1996. From 1993 through 1995, the goal was to complete 145 housing units, but Westside Conservation Corporation completed only 80 units" (Schuldt, 1997a, p. B1).

TABLE 6.4. Westside Conservation Corporation (WCC)'s Housing Performance Data, 1989 to 1994, Housing Unit Performance

Year	Completed	Proposed	% Completed
1989	20	20	100
1990	49	35	140
1991	38	35	108
1992	32	38	84
1993	46	60	76
1994	23	45	51

Source: CBGA (various years)

Despite these problems over the years, the city never pulled WCC's cash advances or terminated its CDBG funding until 1996. The result was that the city lost several hundred thousands of CDBG dollars (Dries, 1996). Instead of penalizing WCC, the city provided an additional $1.4 million in CDBG funds to help it repair properties during the early 1990s. These funds were in addition to the $3.8 million WCC received in new CDBG dollars between 1992 and 1996 (Schuldt, 1997b). Also, the city reacquired forty properties from the agency—fourteen through tax foreclosure. Seventeen others were purchased, repaired, and sold by the city's Community Housing and Preservation Corp (CHPC), and nine were purchased through the Redevelopment Authority of the City of Milwaukee (RACM), which cost the city several hundred thousand additional CDBG dollars (Norman, 1996a; Schuldt, 1997a).

In addition to these forty properties, the city had to raze another thirteen properties owned by WCC, thus costing the city additional CDBG dollars. Moreover, the city expended an additional $47,225 in CDBG funds for the Housing Preservation Corporation to buy three properties formerly owned by the WCC (Schuldt, 1997a). As one Caucasian alderman stated to the outgoing CBGA director at the council's 1997 budget adoption hearing,

> I personally informed you about Westside's troubles several years ago and your office did nothing about them. Now it has cost the city several hundred thousand dollars, the agency has closed, and there are now vacant houses left still needing to be repaired. If your office had acted then, these problems could have been avoided years ago.

This comment was consistent with earlier findings which showed that other city officials were aware of WCC's program performance and fiscal management problems. Although WCC's problems had been known for years, its CDBG funds were not terminated and its Cash Advance was not pulled until 1996. In the end, the city created a special committee to deal with WCC's problems, and it paid portions of the agency's bills to former employees and contractors ("City to use," 1996).

The East Side Housing Action Committee (ESHAC), another Caucasian housing CBO, experienced problems with its CDBG-funded housing programs, but it did not have its CDBG funding cut. ESHAC had legal problems, poor program performance, it experienced major fiscal problems, and it was on the verge of bankruptcy based on its asset/debt ratio. ESHAC kept its cash advance and received several hundred thousand dollars of new CDBG funds (Gordon, personal communication, 1996; Love-Johnson, personal communication, 1997; Norman, 1996d; Norman and Daykin, 1996).

ESHAC experienced additional problems. In January 1996 it was sued by the Housing Partnership Corporation (HPC), a non-profit housing agency, over a $1 million mortgage payment dispute involving twenty-eight single-family and duplex properties ESHAC owned. The suit stated that ESHAC missed $20,357 in payments in 1995 and that it had five outstanding mortgages worth $982,701 owed to it. In 1996, the Milwaukee Housing Assistance Corporation (MHAC) took over the management of eighty of ESHAC's properties (Norman, 1996d). In 1996, the Housing Partnership Corporation foreclosed on twenty-eight properties ESHAC owned. Moreover, ESHAC's management of some properties was so bad that they were taken over by another nonprofit agency, Housing Assistance Corporation, under a court order (Gould, 1996; Norman, 1996d; Norman 1997a). ESHAC's cost reports for its NIPs contained numerous errors, corrections, and adjustments that made it too difficult to process cost reports and to determine the correct amount to pay ESHAC (CBGA, 1993-1997).

Similarly, ESHAC had some problems meeting its housing production program goals. Even with its cash advance, the agency did not meet its housing production goals in any year during the period from 1993 to 1996. The agency did not complete any of its housing units in 1993 (0 percent), and it completed 20 percent in 1994. ESHAC's housing production program during this period did not fare much better than MUFBH, but it retained its cash advance (see Table 6.5). During the period between 1991 and 1995, ESHAC's NIP performance was comparable to the Commandos. In 1991, ESHAC's NIP completed only 63 percent of its scheduled housing units. In other years, it completed 84 to 100 percent of its NIP projects (see Table 6.6.). ESHAC continued to receive CDBG funds while the Commandos lost its CDBG funds.

ESHAC also had problems with its rental property management. In 1997, ESHAC allowed sewage to soak the basement of one of its rental units, resulting in a five-year-old youth becoming very ill and hospitalized with *Giardia,* a parasite transmitted by fecal matter in

TABLE 6.5. ESHAC's Housing Performance Data, 1989 to 1996, Housing Unit Performance

Year	Completed	Proposed	% Completed
1989	6	6	100
1990	14	14	100
1991	11	14	78
1992	18	18	100
1993	0	35	0
1994	6	30	20
1995	30	28	107
1996	7	10	70

Source: CBGA (various years)

water. Another rental tenant's property was flooded and this resulted in the destruction of personal items: family pictures, birth certificates, and other items. Renters' calls to ESHAC for property repairs went unanswered. ESHAC received sixty-six building code violations from the city (Norman, 1997e).

A subcommittee consisting of city representatives (comptroller's office, CBGA office, city attorney's office, common council members and staff) was established to deal with the problems of ESHAC and WCC. A creative approach to addressing ESHAC's problems was to develop a "bailout plan," which was publicly presented as a "marketing plan" to help ESHAC sell its properties to low and moderate-income people per HUD's regulations. ESHAC was provided $117,000 and allowed to keep its cash advance despite the aforementioned problems. The common council's staff and the comptroller's office memo to the CDPC indicated there were too many serious fiscal problems associated with the proposed bailout plan and ESHAC's financial stability (Gordon, personal communication, 1996; Holt, personal communication, 1996). Both the CBGA office and the CDPC were provided this information and were aware of ESHAC's problems, yet approved additional CDBG funding for this CBO.

In addition to the $117,000 in CDBG funds, ESHAC continued to rely on its regular $66,000 cash advance, which it later lost. The common council staff's November 18, 1996, memo further informed the

TABLE 6.6. ESHAC's NIP Performance Data, 1990 to 1995, Housing Unit Performance

Year	Completed	Proposed	% Completed
1990	45	43	104.0
1991	24	38	63.6
1992	38.5	42	91.7
1993	44.5	52	85.6
1994	38	45	84.4
1995	40	40	100.0

Source: CBGA (various years)

CDPC of ESHAC's fiscal problems and legal judgments (Gordon, personal communication, 1996). That memo recommended that ESHAC's cash advance be pulled immediately. Instead of being penalized, ESHAC was allowed to use $45,000 in "new" 1997 CDBG funds and a $25,000 loan from a bank to repay the city for losing the $66,000 cash advance. Despite these problems, ESHAC was provided over $617,843 in new CDBG funds for 1997. ESHAC would later celebrate this bailout (Norman, 1997a; Norman, 1997d; Norman, 1997c). ESHAC's Housing Production Program was never defunded. It withdrew its 1997 CDBG application. The next year ESHAC received an increase in CDBG funds (Nichols, 1998).

NWSCDC is another CDBG-funded Caucasian CBO that experienced fiscal, management, and performance problems. Even though NWSCDC owed over $89,000 in taxes, and it had unaccounted CDBG expenses, the agency was able to continue its cash advance and received new CDBG funding through 1994 to 1997 (Ross, 1994). In 1993, NWSCDC was awarded $40,000 in CDBG funds to acquire a building, demolish it, and pave the landscape at the site. NWSCDC was required to raise another $40,000 in private matching funds, which it failed to raise. It did not complete the project. At its May 1996 meeting, the CDPC waived the requirement that NWSCDC obtain private matching funds and gave NWSCDC an additional year to find money for completion of the parking lot. This extension was granted even though NWSCDC had been awarded the funds several years earlier to do the work and it had not met its contractual goals.

CBGA noted that NWSCDC did not meet its performance goals on another CDBG-funded project. This agency was funded for three years to repair houses as part of a youth employment program, but it did not meet any of its housing production goals. The 1996 CDBG *Briefing Book* noted,

> The program faltered in its three-year history of unit completions. In 1993, 6 units were projected. In 1994, 8 units have been projected. In 1995, 8 units have been projected. As of July 1995, a feasibility package has been submitted for 8 units of housing. Two certificates of occupancy permit for 2 single family units were submitted by applicant. (CBGA, 1996a, p. 240)

These were the same eight housing units carried over from one year to another. Despite these problems, this agency continued to receive CDBG funds and grew into a multimillion dollar agency.

In summary, problematic Caucasian CBOs were often assisted and provided new CDBG funding while African-American CBOs were penalized. African-American CBOs had their cash advances and contracts terminated. They were also denied new CDBG funds, carryover funds, and contract extensions, thus forcing them to close down or scale back their operations. Special subcommittees were not established to assist African-American CBOs, nor were they provided funds to complete the rehabilitation of properties so that the city could meet HUD's requirements of repairing and selling rehabilitation houses to low- and moderate-income residents.

Chapter 7

Bending Existing CDBG Rules

The information gleaned from surveys and extensive reviews of city files revealed that race had an impact when Caucasian or African-American CBOs requested CDBG carryover funds, CDBG contract extensions, and CDBG reprogramming dollars. In a significant number of instances, Caucasian CBOs were granted these privileges while African-American CBOs frequently were denied.

At the end of each year, any unspent CDBG funds went into the CDBG general contingency fund for reallocation purposes that constituted the pool of CDBG reprogramming dollars. This practice occurred unless CBOs requested permission to carryover unspent CDBG funds or to allow that funding to be extended into another year to complete a project. The CBGA staff would receive and review all requests for CDBG carryovers and then forward its recommendations to the CDPC. The willingness to allow CBOs to carryover unspent CDBG dollars was unevenly extended to African-American CBOs. In November 1996, the CDPC adopted a policy that prohibited any CBOs from using carryover funds. Yet several CBOs made carryover requests. Although $127,348 in carryover requests was approved for Caucasian CBOs, no carryover requests from African-American CBOs were approved (see Table 7.1).

The Community Organizing Westside Agency (COWSA), an African-American CBO involved in community organizing activities, had its carryover request of $10,907 denied based on that new policy. This occurred even though the agency received its CDBG late because CBGA signed COWSA's contract late. Southside Community Organization (SCO), a Caucasian CBO involved in community organizing, requested that $10,348 be carried over. That agency's request was approved, even though SCO had received its CDBG funding several months before COWSA.

TABLE 7.1. Requests for 1996 Carryover Funds by CBOs (per $1,000)

CBOs' Race	Request	Approved
AA	293	0
C	857	127
O	14	0
T	1,164	127

Source: CBGA, 1996a
AA = African Americans; C = Caucasians; O = Others; T = Total

Other African-American CBOs had their carryover requests denied while Caucasian CBOs' carryover requests were approved. ESHAC, a Caucasian CBO, whose financial difficulties were discussed earlier in this book was provided $117,000 in carryover funds in the form of an extension. The rationale for these funds was to allow the agency to repair, market, and sell its properties. Meantime, two African-American housing CBOs, Milwaukee United for Better Housing ($159,771) and OIC ($14,160) had their carryover requests denied. MUFBH was not provided any CDBG funds for carryover purposes or extension; and, it had to cease it housing operations.

The decision not to allow African-American CBOs CDBG carryover funds although their requests were similar to Caucasian CBOs and they were being better operated than Caucasian CBOs provides yet another piece of important evidence regarding how Milwaukee allocates and distributes CDBG funds. Race clearly played a factor in deciding which CBOs were allowed to carry over CDBG funds. On one level, these unequal decisions may point to an overt racial animus. Or, they may reflect political alliances and power blocs that are shaped by the realities of Milwaukee's racial inequalities. Either way, African-American CBOs were the losers in this process. Second, the denial of carryover funds affected CBOs' ability to provide services and remain open. The decisions to deny African-American CBOs' requests for carryover funds reduced the amount of CDBG funds going to African-American CBOs and the jobs and services associated with them.

In addition to carryover requests that went before the CDPC in December 1996, the CDPC received requests for contract extensions. A contract extension was granted to complete a project when no new CDBG funds were awarded to an agency next year. As shown in Table 7.2, no African-American CBO had its request for a contract extension approved in December 1996. In one instance, a conditional extension was granted to New Covenant, but this CBO had to submit to an extensive common council and public debate that postponed the award until the spring of 1997. To add insult to injury, the common council cut the allocation from a requested $150,000 to $75,000.

Although the African-American CBO, New Covenant, struggled to get its funding, ESHAC, a Caucasian CBO with highly publicized fiscal, legal, and management problems, was approved for $117,000 in contract extensions using carryover dollars. Throughout Milwaukee's African-American community, residents saw a racially motivated double standard at the simultaneous decisions to grant a special request for ESHAC while forcing New Covenant to endure financial hardship.

African Americans did not fare well when seeking CDBG reprogramming dollars. In June 1997, there were $2.4 million CDBG dollars left from 1996 available for reprogramming purposes. Reprogramming dollars were unspent funds from previous CDBG contracts and CDBG-funded program income. These funds were then reallocated for specific purposes. In 1997, the CBGA created several eligibility criteria for reprogramming dollars. Several eligibility criteria were written so that only city agencies could apply for funding them (Spot Site Acquisition, $746,770; Renewal Site Contingency, $187,000; and the Weed and Seed Program, $107,580) for a total of $1,041,350. This meant that CBOs could only compete for $1,387,021 of the $2,428,371 of CDBG reprogramming dollars. Several CDBG amend-

TABLE 7.2. Requests for 1996 CDBG Contract Extensions by CBOs (per $1,000)

CBOs' Race	Request	Approved
AA	376	0
C	504	160
O	33	0
T	913	160

Source: CBGA, 1996a
AA = African Americans; C = Caucasians; O = Others; T = Total

ments, totaling $72,735, were passed at the CDBG reprogramming hearing for various projects sponsored by Caucasian CBOs. CDBG contingency funds were used for those amended projects.

Initially, the data showed that African-American CBOs were the winners in the allocation of 1996 CDBG reprogramming dollars. African-American CBOs received $738,158 in reprogramming dollars and 70.9 percent of their requests were approved. Caucasian CBOs received $682,850 in 1996 reprogramming dollars and had 44 percent of their reprogramming proposals approved (see Table 7.3).

Although the initial data show that African-American CBOs fared well during the awarding of CDBG reprogramming dollars, it does not tell the story behind those numbers and how African Americans were disadvantaged in this process. One African-American CBO, Carpenter's Incorporated, a housing agency, was awarded $370,000 in CDBG reprogramming dollars after it was denied funding several months earlier for alleged performance problems. The city's CBGA director provided the common council and the CDPC with inaccurate and incomplete information on its performance. When the reprogramming allocation was made with surplus CDBG funds, Carpenters Incorporated had already suffered an unjust turn: it had lost funding despite exceeding its contractual goals.

As is common with CBOs working in economically depressed areas, the temporary loss of funding is enough to destabilize the organization and create the conditions for its closure or failure. Despite the $370,000 reprogramming award, Carpenter's Incorporated was never able to receive or spend the money. Once again, many in Milwaukee's African-American community were angered by the city govern-

TABLE 7.3. CDBG 1996 Reprogramming Dollars Awarded to CBOs by Agency Race

CBO's Race	Request	Approved
AA	1,040	738
C	1,532	682
O	46	39
T	2,618	1,459

Source: CBGA, 1996a
AA = African Americans; C = Caucasians; O = Others; T = Total

ment's claim that this $370,000 award was an instance of helping an African-American CBO.

Besides obscuring the story behind the Carpenter's Incorporated case, the listing of the CDBG reprogramming awards did not reveal how criteria were written to give certain groups an advantage when applying for funds. One criterion for eligibility for CDBG reprogramming funds was that a group must have been awarded $1 during the CDBG regular funding cycle, the previous fall. Seven CBOs were awarded $1 during the CDPC regular allocation cycle, several months earlier. These included five Caucasian CBOs (NWSCDC, Milwaukee Christian Center, LAND, Agape, and Act Landmark Housing) and two African-American CBOs (Carpenter's Incorporated and MUFBH). Four of the five Caucasian CBOs (NWSCDC, Milwaukee Christian Center, LAND, Agape) were funded during the CDBG reprogramming cycle for a total of $126,569. The only Caucasian agency awarded $1, which was not provided CDBG Reprogramming dollars, was ACT Landmark Housing, which was ineligible for CDBG funds. In contrast, only one (Carpenter's Incorporated) of the two African-American CBOs was provided CDBG reprogramming dollars, but city officials already knew that it was never in a position to use those funds. Once again, the evidence pointed to decisions that rewarded Caucasian CBOs at the expense of African-American CBOs.

The CDBG reprogramming allocation also does not tell the story regarding the three amendments made to the CBGA's reprogramming recommendations that showed how African-American CBOs were treated differently. All three recommendations involved Caucasian CBOs. One amendment provided $20,000 to ESHAC for a home buyer counseling program. ESHAC was not eligible for those funds based on the CDBG reprogramming criteria approved by the CDPC. But these CDBG funds were awarded, and at a time when ESHAC's fiscal and management problems were highly publicized in the local press and the agency was on the verge of bankruptcy. All the CDBG funds scheduled for CDBG reprogramming purposes had been allocated, which meant the $20,000 would eventually come from the CDBG contingency fund.

Another CDBG reprogramming amendment provided Journey House (a Caucasian CBO) $37,584 for funding to market a targeted investment neighborhood (TIN) on the city's south side. Several problems existed with this amendment. Based on the CDBG reprogramming criteria, this project was not eligible for CDBG funds. All the available CDBG reprogramming funds had been allocated for other projects. This meant that some projects would have to be reduced or another funding source would have to be found. Finally, the CDBG program had not funded the marketing of TINs in the past. Instead, it provided CDBG funding for actual work (land clearance, repair of housing) of TINs.

The third reprogramming amendment related to increasing the Nonprofit Center's recommended amount from $27,549 to $42,700, an increase of $15,151, or more than 50 percent. This increase was approved even though the CBGA had made a policy that certain personnel expenses incurred before July 1997 would be ineligible for CDBG reprogramming dollars. No other CBO seeking CDBG funds for similar personnel activities was approved during this period.

Other federal funds were awarded by the CDPC during the regular CDBG allocation process. The HOME Program, a federally-funded housing program, received such funds. The city allocated these funds using a formula-based method. The HOME Program is a federally funded housing initiative created by the National Affordable Housing Act of 1990. The HOME Program is designed to provide funding to expand the supply of decent, safe, sanitary, and affordable housing (primarily rental); to strengthen the abilities of state and local governments to provide housing; and to assure that federal housing services, financing, and other investments are provided to state and local governments in a coordinated, supportive fashion (ICF Incorporated, 1992).

The city awarded HOME funds to housing groups that received CDBG funds using a per-unit formula, whereby $15,000 per unit was awarded to housing groups awarded CDBG funds. In 1996, the city awarded more than $7 million in HOME funds to housing groups for 1997 housing activities (Skiba, personal communication, 1997). Table 7.4 shows that African-American housing groups' share of HOME funds decreased significantly between 1993 and 1997 from a high of 29.4 percent in 1993 to only 9 percent in 1997.

Awarding these HOME funds through the CDBG RFP process worked to the disadvantage of African-American CBOs in several ways. The various CBOs do not have any input into deciding how those funds were being used since they were awarded on a formula basis, rather than need. Since the quality of housing in the African-

TABLE 7. 4. Home Funds to CBOs by Race (per $1,000)

Year	CBOs' Race			
	AA	**C**	**O**	**T**
1993	1,655	3,967	0	5,622
1994	1,365	3,600	75	5,040
1995	1,275	4,345	80	5,700
1996	1,005	5,486	120	6,611
1997	405	4,065	0	4,470
T	5,705	21,463	275	27,443

Source: CBGA (various groups)

AA = African Americans; C = Caucasians; O = Others; T = Total

American community was much older and more deteriorated than other parts of the city, it required more funding per unit than was allowed by the formula. When African-American housing CBOs were defunded, they not only lost their CDBG funds but they lost their HOME funds as well. This further reduced the amount of federal funds going to African-American CBOs. Moreover, the awarding of other CDBG funds with little public scrutiny limited the amount of funds potentially awarded to African-American CBOs.

Existing CDBG rules and practices were bent to assist ineligible Caucasian CBOs receiving CDBG funds while denying funding for eligible African-American CBOs. The CBGA required that a CBO have a two-year successful "track record" performing the proposed activity. CBGA's guidelines stated that any agency receiving CDBG funds must be incorporated and have provided program services for two years prior to receiving CDBG funds or show evidence of broad-based support or matching funds. CBOs had to demonstrate that they were financially viable, and that they would be able to maintain a minimal level of program activity even without CDBG funds (CBGA, 1991). Generally, an agency was considered to be a nonprofit group if it had a 501(c) status and documentation (a Letter of Determination) from the Internal Revenue Services (IRS). If a CBO lacked the two-year track record, the CBGA could make a policy exception, if the CBO had a fiscal agent, an established CBO, to manage the project until the group became eligible for CDBG funds.

The CBGA clearly violated its own policy when it recommended $70,000 in CDBG funds and $150,000 in HOME funds for a Caucasian CBO (ACT Landmark), even though that group was ineligible for CDBG funds based on its existing criteria. ACT Landmark's proposal clearly showed that it was ineligible for CDBG funds. This CBO was incorporated in May 1996, one month before the deadline for submitting 1997 CDBG applications, and it did not have a Letter of Determination from the IRS indicating that it was a nonprofit agency. This CBO's revenue was clearly insufficient to perform housing production activities. It had revenue of $5,000 in 1995 and $35,000 in 1996, which was insufficient to pay for the repair of one housing unit. Finally, the agency did not have a fiscal agent to oversee its operations until it became eligible for CDBG funds.

Even though the CBGA was aware of this group's ineligibility, it still recommended $220,000 in CDBG and home funding. The mayor indicated in a meeting with his CDPC representative, the CBGA director, the CDPC vice-chair, and the common council's staff that he wanted this group funded in 1997. The mayor stated that he wanted this CBO funded because it was not part of a religious coalition called MICAH, and he thought it had been doing some good things in its targeted area. The CBGA director was unsuccessful in his effort to get this group funded at the CDPC. The common council's staff prepared a written analysis to the CDPC that revealed that this group was ineligible for CDBG and HOME funds based on the aforementioned reasons. Although this CBO was ineligible for CDBG funds, the mayor's CDPC representative got $1 of CDBG funds awarded to it at the zoning, neighborhoods, and development committee (ZN&D), which made the group eligible for the $150,000 in HOME funds that the CBGA had recommended. The CDPC vice-chair informed the CBGA that he did not want a group that was given $1 in CDBG funds to be eligible for $150,000 in HOME funds. The CBGA, then under a new director, agreed with the CDPC vice-chair's view, and it did not provide this group any CDBG or HOME funds.

Although the CBGA was trying to award CDBG funds to an ineligible Caucasian CBO, it recommended $0 in funding for an African-American CBO, Fighting Back Initiative, which was involved in community organizing. CBGA stated that this group was ineligible for CDBG funds because it was not incorporated. This claim was disputable. This group had been in existence for several years and it was in the process of getting its Letter of Determination indicating that it was a tax-exempt CBO. More importantly, the agency had a fiscal agent, the Social Development Commission (SDC), overseeing the project. This should have met the CBGA's requirements for having a fiscal agent. This CBO was not recommended for CDBG funds.

Once again, race clearly played a role in deciding which CBO seeking funding for the first time was recommended for CDBG funds. In this case, an African-American CBO was recommended for no funding although it had a fiscal agent, and it had been in existence for several years. In contrast, the ACT Landmark was incorporated one month before the CDBG proposal deadline, it had no fiscal agent, it did not have a Letter of Determination showing that it was a tax-exempt agency, and it lacked resources to perform the proposed activities.

The CBGA altered its rules again for a Caucasian CBO in awarding CDBG funds to administer a revolving loan program, whereby a CBO was provided CDBG funds to make loans. An African-American CBO, Martin Luther King (MLK) Incorporation, sought $75,000 to operate a revolving loan program for making loans to minority businesses. The CBGA recommended no funding for this project. The CBGA director, at the time, indicated to the common council's staff that the CBGA did not award revolving loan funds to any CBOs (Brady, personal communication, 1996). The MLK agency did not receive any CDBG funds for that program. However, the CBGA recommended $150,000 for a revolving loan project operated by Family Services of Milwaukee, a Caucasian CBO. This program made loans to low-income people who had exhausted all their loan options, and whom also had little or no collateral. The CDPC eventually approved Family Services' proposal, but at a reduced level, $90,000. Once again, these findings offered empirical evidence to support the claim that African Americans were not receiving their fair share of Milwaukee's CDBG funds.

Chapter 8

Conclusion:
How Race Directly Affects
the Allocation of CDBG Funds
in Milwaukee

The interviews, surveys, and analysis of CDBG documents, trace analysis of CDBG proposals, participant observations, and analysis of other supporting documents all support the idea that the mayor was the dominant figure in the CDBG allocation process for several reasons. One, the mayor made the initial CDBG funding recommendations. Once the mayor's CDBG recommendations were made, they were seldom changed, especially during Mayor Norquist's administrations. This pattern had significant implications for the allocation of CDBG funds to African-American neighborhoods and African-American CBOs. Two, the mayor appointed the director of the CBGA, which oversaw, monitored, and evaluated the operation of the CDBG program. The CBGA worked for the mayor and pursued his agenda. This affected the evaluation of CBOs' CDBG proposals and CDBG funding recommendations. Three, the mayor had veto power over CDBG-funded categories. If the mayor vetoed a CBO's CDBG funding, the common council needed a two-thirds vote (twelve of seventeen votes) to override the veto. This was a serious problem for African-American council members since they were only five of seventeen councilors. Finally, CBOs recognized that the mayor was the most powerful figure in the CDBG funding process for the reasons previously cited. As a result, these groups did not speak out against the mayor/CBGA in CDBG funding decisions for fear of losing their CDBG funding.

Although the two mayors in this study took different approaches with the use of CDBG funds, the result was the same: racial considerations appeared to be a factor in the distribution of CDBG funds in Milwaukee. Under Mayor Maier, the city used a large share of its CDBG funds for capital improvement projects (CIPs) throughout the city in early years, but mostly in African-American areas in later years. This use of CDBG funds impacted the African-American community negatively in several ways. CDBG funds intended to eliminate blight and poverty, mostly concentrated in the city's African-American community, were now being used for CIPs. CDBG funds were being used to supplant rather than supplement tax-levy funds for CIPs. Instead of using both CDBG funds and the tax-levy funds for CIPs and having a greater impact in the African-American community, CDBG funds were being used for CIPs. By using CDBG funds for CIPs, CDBG dollars available for other CDBG categories (public services, housing, economic development projects) where African Americans had greater needs, were now limited. Likewise, the use of CDBG dollars for CIPs kept those funds under the direct control of municipal agencies and out of neighborhoods. City agencies dominated by Caucasians had control over those CDBG funds, and they controlled the jobs and subcontracts associated with them. This further limited African Americans' access to and their input into how city agencies used those CDBG funds. The use of CDBG dollars to perform CIPs rather than perform other services resulted in a diminishing impact on the city's African-American community.

African-American CBOs experienced a decline in all three major funding categories (economic development, housing, and public services) between 1988 and 1997 under the popular Caucasian liberal Mayor Norquist's administrations. African-American CBOs suffered drastic funding cuts in all housing categories (housing production, housing rehabilitation, housing production-others, HOME) which resulted in them losing millions of CDBG and HOME dollars. In an effort to keep the city's tax rate low, the mayor used several millions of CDBG dollars to pay for city services and jobs previously funded by tax-levy dollars. This resulted in a growing number of services and jobs being shifted out of the CDBG funding categories and directly administered through the city government. This translated into yet another direct dilution of the ability of African Americans to use the CDBG funds as a means of strengthening their CBOs and communities.

This study also raised serious questions regarding the notion of African-American political empowerment in explaining public allocation distribution patterns. Proponents of racial politics argued that as the number of African-American elected officials increased, the African-American community would receive an increase in benefits, which was not the case in Milwaukee. There was a reduction in the percentage and amount of CDBG funds going to African-American CBOs and African-American neighborhoods. This study revealed that the increasing number of African-American elected officials did not result in more CDBG benefits to African-American neighborhoods and African-American CBOs, raising concerns about the merits of racial political assumptions for several reasons.

These assumptions did not consider that an increase in the number of African-American elected officials might actually create other problems. They competed among themselves for the role of "the African-American leader" or wanted to get the "credit" for a project, which resulted in them being split on policy issues, or undermining other African-American council members' program initiatives.

Also, the racial politics proponents failed to recognize that there were structural limitations (mayor's veto power, biased city agencies, entrenched bureaucracies) on African-Americans' political power. City agencies' practices, which appeared race neutral on the surface, were having negative impacts on African-American CBOs.

Likewise, some African-American members missed key CDPC hearings during critical votes on which the fate of major African-American housing projects and their CDBG funds were at stake. For instance, one African-American council member, missed a key vote to attend a nonmandatory out-of-state conference. This person sent his legislative assistant to the CDPC on his behalf, even though his aide's presence did not have any impact on the committee's decision.

Moreover, African-American officials did not vote along racial lines on CDBG issues. They tended to vote individually rather than as a political voting bloc. Sometimes, they voted against other African-American council members' projects. This situation further reduced their political clout.

In addition, African-American elected officials had different levels of CDPC involvement. While some sought benefits for their districts, others just responded to the CDBG agenda items. In eighteen months of participant observation, African-Americans on the CDPC did not propose any major CDBG policy initiatives. Some African-American council members were concerned with one or two "pet" CDBG projects, but showed little or no interest in other aspects of the CDBG program.

Similar to Caucasian council members, African-American council members voted to shift CDBG funding to citywide projects and city departments as a means of keeping the city's tax rate down, even if it meant less CDBG funds were available for their aldermanic districts.

Furthermore, this study revealed that African-American political power diminished as public policy issues moved through the legislative process. Though African-American councilors had more clout at the committee level on the CPDC, their statistical minority on the common council left them without the power to approve CDBG projects at the full council level, or to override the mayor on final CDBG allocation decisions. Though the relatively high number of African Americans serving on the CPDC gave the impression of representation, it had little or no real effect when the full common council had to make a decision. All too often, African-American councilors were isolated and divided against themselves when it came to mounting a credible challenge to the Caucasian council majority or the administrations of Mayor Maier and Mayor Norquist.

African-American councilors on the CDPC did not demand a greater level of respect from the CBGA. They allowed the CBGA to provide them with agenda items and other crucial information needed to make informed CDBG-funding decisions at the last minute: a day before the meeting, a few hours before the meeting, or during CDPC meetings. These practices would not have been accepted by Caucasian councilors, nor would the CBGA have attempted these practices. Even in this regard, race matters!

Finally, African-American councilors did not use their legislative powers or provide vocal opposition to questionable CBGA policies and practices. They did not hold the CBGA and other city agencies that received CDBG funds accountable for their use of CDBG funds and their treatment of African-American CBOs.

Proponents of racial politics downplayed the instability and changing nature of biracial political coalitions between African-American elected and Caucasian elected officials. Under Mayor Norquist's administrations, African-American CBOs were increasingly eliminated from the CDBG program. African-American CBOs witnessed a drastic decrease in their share of CDBG funds. Furthermore, the mayor and his administration, including the CBGA, were very skillful. They co-opted and diffused attempts to create a biracial coalition to challenge CDBG funding decisions by threatening to reduce or eliminate CBOs' CDBG funding. Mayor Norquist's CDPC representative would later publicly confirm this pattern of intimidation and threats in a sexual harassment lawsuit against him that generated considerable public debate.

Although some liberal Caucasian public officials in Milwaukee supported African-American elected officials and CBOs on some non-controversial issues, those same Caucasian public officials were not always willing to support them on high-profile and controversial issues that could put them in direct conflict with other powerful Caucasian elected officials or interest groups. Those Caucasian officials would have risked their political support if they supported African-American elected officials and African-American CBOs on high-profile and controversial matters. Also, some of the leading critics of African-American CBOs were liberal Caucasian common council members who had some of the worst performing CDBG-funded groups, especially in the housing areas, located in their aldermanic districts. These liberal Caucasian common council members voted to eliminate or reduce African-American CBOs' funding on a regular basis. Finally, Caucasian council members competed against African-American council members for CDBG funding for their aldermanic districts. When this occurred, political biracial coalitions took a back seat to their desires to obtain CDBG funding for their aldermanic districts.

Racial politics proponents failed to realize that public bureaucracies were not independent government agencies. Instead, they were an extension of the mayor's office as was the case of the CBGA. As mentioned earlier, the mayor appointed the CBGA director, who served at the mayor's pleasure. The CBGA director hired the CBGA staff. The CBGA oversaw, monitored, and evaluated the operation of the CDBG program. The CBGA worked for the mayor and pursued his agenda, which affected the evaluation of CBOs' CDBG proposals and CDBG funding recommendations. Moreover, the CBGA controlled the volume and quality of information on the CDBG program needed to make informed CDBG policy decisions and allocation decisions. CBOs provided all CDBG-related documents to the CBGA, which made the CBGA the gatekeeper of that information. CBGA approved or disapproved CBOs' proposed expenditures via their cost reports. This had significant consequences for CBOs' hiring and contracting practices. If the mayor or CBGA did not want someone hired by a CBO as an employee or contractor, CBGA did not have to approve that cost as an appropriate CDBG expenditure. The CBGA staffed the CDPC, prepared the CDPC members' CDBG agendas and books, prepared group performance reports, and other relevant documents. The CBGA determined the quality and timeliness of CDBG information provided to CDPC members for their review, which limited the CDPC members' role because many times they did not have adequate time to review these materials. Likewise, until 1996 the CDPC did not have its own independent staff person to review and analyze CDBG proposals and related materials that CBGA provided. The CDPC members were dependent on the mayor's staff to provide complete, accurate, and unbiased CDBG information, which was not always the case. African-American CBOs were more likely than Caucasian CBOs to lose their funding or have their cash advances terminated when they experienced problems. In the area of housing production, by 1997, all African-American housing producers had been defunded, whereas Caucasian CBOs with similar or worse problems remained funded. Moreover, when African-American CBOs had cost overruns, they were denied CDBG funding (Genesis project) or had their CDBG funding stalled and later reduced (New Covenant). At the same time, Caucasian CBOs such as WCC, NWSCDC, and ESHAC were provided new CDBG funds, despite their problems. African-Americans CBOs experiencing problems (program operation, fiscal problems, and financial problems) were held to higher performance standards than were Caucasian CBOs with similar or worse problems.

Successful African-American CDBG programs had their funding cut or eliminated. CDBG programs (SDC, Commandos, Carpenter's Incorporated) were penalized under Mayor Norquist's administrations via inaccurate and biased write-ups, while poorly operated Caucasian CBOs (ESHAC, NWSCDC, WCC) flourished and grew into multimillion dollar CBOs. Although the mayor was willing to veto funding for a successfully operated African-American CBO (SDC), he was not willing to take such action against problematic Caucasian CBOs. The CBGA did not provide technical assistance or establish a special committee to problematic African-American CBOs as was done with ESHAC and WCC in 1996. In addition, problematic Caucasian CBOs did not reach the full common council for public debate as was the case of New Covenant and SDC projects. Finally, CBGA bent its existing policies to assist ineligible Caucasian CBOs to receive CDBG funds while denying eligible African-American CBOs CDBG funds.

The comptroller's practice of pulling CBOs' cash advances appeared to be biased against African-American CBOs. The decision to rescind a CBO's cash advance was applied differently toward African-American CBOs and Caucasian CBOs that resulted in African-American CBOs not meeting their CDBG performance goals, which in turn resulted in their contracts being reduced or terminated. Since many groups counted on the cash advance for operating purposes until their CDBG funds or other funding became available, the elimination of the cash advance resulted in them reducing or halting their CDBG-funded activities. This then contributed to their performance problems, thus giving the city ammunition to reduce or eliminate their funding. This study showed that when African-American CBOs experienced performance or financial problems, the comptroller's office pulled their cash advances immediately as in the case of the Commandos, O. C. White Soul Club, and other African-American CBOs. Meanwhile, problematic Caucasian groups such as WCC, ESHAC, and NWSCDC kept and lost their cash advance.

CDBG allocation patterns in Milwaukee also indicated that community need was a minimal factor in the distribution of these federal dollars for several reasons. CDBG funds were allocated based on administrative funding categories, and not targeted toward geographic areas based on need. The CDBG boundaries have changed over the years and have been expanded outward from the core of the city, where the worse socioeconomic conditions have existed. Furthermore, the 1997 change to the CDBG allocation process expanded the CDBG boundaries even farther, causing most of the CDBG boundaries to cover almost the entire city's boundary. Similarly, the city's increasing share of CDBG funds, and its creation of citywide funding categories diluted the amount of CDBG funds available for the city's neediest areas, which were predominately African-American.

Moreover, the data revealed that although some CDBG dollars were going to African-American aldermanic districts, a large share of those dollars were being awarded to Caucasian CBOs (ESHAC, LAND, NWSCDC, Sherman Park Community Association, YMCA, YWCA, and NHS) located in those districts. In none of the Caucasian aldermanic districts did African-American CBOs receive a large share of CDBG funds. The defunding of African-American CBOs resulted in Caucasian CBOs (Sherman Park, YWCA, ESHAC, and Milwaukee Christian Center) taking on their duties. These Caucasian CBOs had less ties and commitment to the community being served, thus reducing their performance and advocacy. When African-American CBOs were defunded, they lost control of those CDBG dollars. This had a significant impact on hiring decisions since African-American CBOs were more likely to hire other African Americans than were Caucasian CBOs. In a city such as Milwaukee, it is important to have African-American CBOs available to employ African Americans. The defunding of African-American CBOs further affected their ability to subcontract with other African-American businesses. As this study revealed, the share of African-American businesses receiving subcontracting dollars from CBOs decreased significantly as African-American CBOs were defunded. This further limited the growth of some African-American businesses.

Although this study has tried to point out the structural and institutional reasons for these inequalities, African-American CBOs must take some of the blame for allowing these actions to occur. There were vested interests in African-American CBOs within the African-American community that also benefited from, and sought to protect the status quo of CDBG funding allocation decisions. They were allies of Caucasian elected officials and were not willing to jeopardize such relationships. These "vested interests" publicly supported CDBG policies that were detrimental to the African-American community as a whole in exchange for limited CDBG funds for their favorite CBOs. They either did not understand the broader picture of CDBG policies and their implications or they sold out to advance their own selfish interests. As a result, the African-American community as a whole suffered.

Furthermore, the CDBG funding process revealed that African-American CBOs were not as vocal, organized, and united as Caucasian CBOs in opposing CDBG-funding decisions. During the summer of 1997 when the mayor's office/CBGA implemented a new CDBG allocation system for 1998, controversy arose when $660,000 in CDBG funds were shifted from the north side of the city (mostly African Americans) to the south side (mostly Caucasians). There was little organized opposition to that move by African-American CBOs. When those funds were shifted back to the north side, there were over 200 residents from the south side at the CDPC hearing to protest this shift. When the full common council later voted to shift the funds back from the north side to the south side, CBO representatives and residents from the south side were in attendance. There was virtually no representation from north-side residents or African-American CBOs.

Supporters of the racial politics perspective overestimated the level of political involvement and political interest in the growing African-American community. Proponents of racial politics believed that as the percentage of African Americans increases in a community, they become more informed and active in politics. Yet this perspective did not recognize that the growth in Milwaukee's African-American community came from the most impoverished, politically inactive and isolated segment. In a growing African-American community such as Milwaukee, which rates very high on virtually every social and economic problem, the African-American community might actually be less politically active and informed. It is very difficult for impoverished individuals to be interested in politics, let alone CDBG decisions, when they struggle to survive daily.

On the other extreme, some African-American professionals and African-American middle class residents were not willing to jeopardize their status positions to "rock the boat" relative to politics in general, and CDBG funds in particular. In addition, some African-American elected officials, public bureaucrats, middle-class residents, professionals, and "vested interest groups," who understood the CDBG issues, were not willing to jeopardize their privileged positions by challenging the CDBG allocation practices raised in this study. They would privately discuss these matters, but would not discuss them publicly. The racial politics perspective underestimated the division within the African-American community that undermined its progress. They assumed that the African-American community was homogenous and united when it came to social and political change, which was not the case.

This study demonstrated the importance of examining decision-making processes that resulted in funding outcomes using qualitative methods. Often, researchers focus on the outcome of policy decisions rather than the processes used to arrive at those decisions. It was imperative to examine the decision-making process for several reasons. By studying the decision-making processes, students of racial politics can learn how, and to what degree, race plays a role. Students can identify where crucial funding decisions were made, how they affected African-American CBOs, and how other factors and actors were involved in those decision-making processes. They can learn how rules were made and applied toward different groups (Caucasian CBOs versus African-American CBOs) and their funding implications. By studying the decision-making process as opposed to the outcome, students can also learn who did not get funded, and why those groups were not funded. By using qualitative methods, the role of race was revealed more so than when quantitative tools were used. Quantitative data did not tell the entire story that goes with the numbers. Although quantitative data provided valuable information on how much was received and by whom, the data did not provide information on how those funding decisions were made, the process used, and factors that determined the amount received. Qualitative tools (review of performance reports, mail surveys, telephone interviews, in-person interviews, census data, and maps) provided insights into how race affected racial politics. The in-person interviews with public officials and CBO representatives provided insight into how race affected the CDBG funding process that could not be captured by merely using quantitative measures. The use of qualitative measures such as trace analysis allowed the examination of the decision-making process and the determination of how one component of the process affected another part. Eligibility criteria, which appeared race neutral, were established at one point in the decision-making process (eligibility for CDBG reprogramming funds), but later had negative racial consequences in another part of the process.

For these reasons, African Americans' share of CDBG funds will continue to decline unless the quality of African-American council members and African-American CBOs improves, and the CDBG funding allocation process becomes race neutral. African-American council members must learn the importance of unity and voting as a racial bloc, maintain racial coalition building, and better understand CBGA's structural operation and the CDBG allocation process. African-American councilors must be able and willing to hold Caucasian CBOs to the same performance and accountability standards to which African-American CBOs are held. Furthermore, as long as problematic Caucasian CBOs such as ESHAC, WCC, and NWSCDC are able to keep their cash advances and receive new CDBG contracts while African-American groups such as the Commandos, Carpenters, and SDC lose their CDBG contracts and cash advances, racial inequities will continue in the CDBG funding process.

The CDBG funding trends appear even less promising for the city's African-American community based on recent trends. A 1998 change to Milwaukee's CDBG allocation process provides for an even bleaker outlook as CBOs will now be required to "sell" their services rather than be given an outright CDBG grant. Given the racial segregation and racial problems in the city, African-American CBOs will have a hard time selling their services to Caucasian areas, resulting in less CDBG funds for them. This decline might cause some CBOs to reduce their services or cease their operations. Under this new process, a portion of CDBG funds and HOME funds ($501,000) was allocated to majority Caucasian areas outside the CDBG current boundaries. This further reduced funds for African-American areas. Likewise, as a result of the 1998 CDBG reforms, city government allocated several millions of dollars directly to its own agencies in an effort to bolster its finances and pay for existing and additional services. The new funding process allowed for a transfer of millions of dollars in CDBG funds without a need for the submission of proposals through the CPDC and other existing review mechanisms. Besides limiting public scrutiny and debate, this shift in CDBG funding resulted in limiting the amount of CDBG funds available for African-American CBOs. The 1998 reforms allowed city agencies to bid for funding to provide services in the seventeen neighborhood strategic planning areas. Obviously, this increased city agencies' share of CDBG funds at the expense of neighborhood-based CBOs.

As long as the current mayor seeks to continue to provide the city with a lower tax rate, another source of nonproperty tax revenue will be needed. As the largest pool of nonproperty tax revenue given to the city on an annual basis, CDBG funds are the most likely source for offsetting a reduced tax rate.

Inconsistent levels of involvement, lack of public scrutiny, and racial biases contributed to unequal treatment in the CDBG allocation process. These unequal CDBG allocation patterns have resulted in the decline of CDBG funds to African-American communities and

CBOs, thus contributing to their further decline. Rather than eliminate the poverty and blight in the African-American community via CDBG allocations, the city's CDBG allocation patterns and their corresponding impacts might have actually contributed to a decline in Milwaukee's African-American neighborhoods via increased poverty, a declining housing stock, and blight. Although public debate often attributed the decline of African-American areas to the loss of manufacturing jobs, white flight, a declining tax base, and other macroeconomic issues, a dialogue on how the city's CDBG allocation patterns have contributed to the African-American community's social and economic ills should be conducted. In spite of the over $247 million in federal CDBG funds that the city received during this study period, the impact on the African-American community has been relatively minor. In the end, although the federal government was providing CDBG funds to the city to help deal with problems faced by areas such as the city's African-American communities, the city did not use the CDBG funds for their intended purposes.

Appendix A

Research Methods

The city of Milwaukee was used as a case study to examine the allocation of CDBG funds and to determine what role race plays in that process. A case study can be defined as an in-depth, multifaceted investigation, using qualitative research methods to analyze a single social phenomenon. It allows for an empirical inquiry of a phenomenon within its real-life context (Feagin et al., 1991; Merriam, 1990; Patton, 1990; Yin, 1994).

The case study approach offers several advantages. It allows for researchers to study human events and their actions in a natural setting, and it retains a holistic approach, thus providing meaningful data on real-life events such as individual life cycles and organizational cycles. Furthermore, the case study approach captures people as they experience their daily routines, providing researchers with valuable empirical and theoretical insights into understanding larger social complexes. A case study further permits the researcher to examine not only the complexity of life in which people find themselves, but the impact of beliefs and decisions on the complex web of social actions. The case study enables a researcher to examine the flow of social life over time and to display the patterns of everyday life as they change. A case study permits the researcher to uncover the historical dimension of a societal phenomenon or setting. Finally, it allows for development of propositions that can be used for the generation of new ideas and social science theories (Feagin et al., 1991; Merriam, 1990; Yin, 1994).

The case study method also has its limitations. Case studies do not focus on the relationship between variables, as do quantitative approaches (Feagin et al., 1991). The case study approach has also been criticized for its lack of rigor. Yin (1994, p. 9) states,

> Perhaps the greatest concern has been over the lack of rigor of case study investigation. Too many times, the case study investigation has been sloppy and has allowed equivocal evidence of biased views to influence the direction of the findings and conclusion.

The case study does not allow for generalization since it focuses on a unique setting, thus it makes it difficult to generalize the study's findings from one setting to another. Finally, the case study has been criticized for being time-consuming and resulting in the collection of too much useless data (Yin, 1994).

In this study, data sources were used to determine the distribution of CDBG funding and its impact on the city's African-American community and CBOs. Specifically, the study relied on published CDBG proposals, city files, and other public materials (Grantee Performance Reports, CDPC Minutes, etc.) for the years 1975 to 1997. This included the Ollie reports, internal documents prepared by the Community Block Grant Administration (CBGA) that listed every agency receiving CDBG funds in a given year by category, and how much CDBG funding was recommended at each of the CDBG funding stage. The Ollie reports were used for the years between 1988 to 1997. The original goal was to collect data on all CDBG proposals from 1975 to 1997, the entire CDBG funding period in Milwaukee. Since some of the early years' data were missing, this study was forced to select five-year intervals: 1975, 1980, 1985, 1990, and 1995 to make the data from Mayor Maier's and Mayor Norquist's years comparable. More complete and consecutive years' data were used for Mayor Norquist's years (1988 to 1997). The focus was on the three largest categories (housing, economic development, and public services) for which CBOs received CDBG funds.

A second major methodological approach was to survey a variety of reports and data sources outside of municipal government, particularly articles from local newspapers (*Milwaukee Journal Sentinel, Milwaukee Courier,* and the *Milwaukee Community Journal*) and studies published in academic journals, books, and special reports.

Face-to-face interviews were conducted with key elected officials, public bureaucrats, and CBOs' representatives involved in the CDBG program. The goals in these open-ended interviews were to obtain detailed background information on the CDBG program, its politics, and data on the distribution of CDBG funds which could not be gleaned from quantitative methods. A total of twenty-one individuals were interviewed, which included fifteen former or present elected officials and six former or present city administrators. Three individuals (one former common council member and two former public bureaucrats) declined my requests to interview them. Interviews were conducted during the months of July 1994 and August 1994, and they were conducted in a variety of settings (government buildings, CBO offices, and at a public park). Seventeen interviews were done in person with no tape recording, three interviews were taped, and one interview was conducted over the telephone. Interviews lasted from twenty to forty-five minutes.

Besides interviews, confidential surveys were mailed to fifty CBOs that had received at least two consecutive years of CDBG funding between 1975 and 1994 to obtain information on the CDBG program and their perspectives on it. CBOs' names were obtained from CDBG proposals and other CDBG reports. CBOs were chosen randomly from these data sources. A total of twenty-four surveys were returned after two mailings. Seven returned surveys could not be used because some CBOs were no longer in existence or did not want to participate in the study. Thus, seventeen out of a possible twenty-four returned surveys were useable.

CBOs were asked to exclude their identity from the surveys and the self-addressed return envelopes that were provided. No codes were included on the surveys that would have enabled responding CBOs to be identified, which may have jeopardized their funding. It is not known which CBOs completed and returned the surveys. Returned CBOs' surveys were named as follows: CBO-A, CBO-B, and so forth based on the order they were returned. All CBO surveys were mailed and returned in 1994.

A "trace analysis" approach was also used in this study. Using this procedure, CDBG proposals were traced through each CDBG funding decision-making step (CBGA/mayor's, CDPC, common council's committees) to determine where funding decisions were changed, and the types of agencies impacted by them. For Mayor Maier's years (1975-1976, 1980-1981, and 1985-1986), the Community Development Program Annual Evaluation Report was used, which provided data on the CBOs that applied for, and received CDBG funding, along with other CDBG documents. It also listed CBOs recommended for funding by CDBG program category and the amount recommended at each funding level.

In 1996, I was hired by the CDPC as an independent consultant, which later became a city position (CDBG fiscal analyst) to evaluate CDBG proposals, make CDBG funding recommendations, and conduct fiscal research and public policy analyses on CDBG-related issues. Likewise, I provided written and oral reports to the CDPC on a regular basis. This new position afforded me a unique insider's look at the CDBG funding process, one typically not available to outsiders nor captured by quantitative outcome measures. I took advantage of my position to become a participant observer of the inner workings of the CDBG funding process. This unique point of view has provided me with the ability to uncover hidden practices in which race forges the distribution of urban services.

Other data sources were obtained as follows. The aldermanic districts that CBOs resided in were identified by obtaining addresses from the CDBG proposals and other CBGA documents. The addresses were then matched with aldermanic districts by using the city's Election Commission Audit of Polling Place Card reports, which listed the addresses of streets by aldermanic districts. The alderperson's race was identified either through my own personal knowledge of him or her, or through discussions with other people who knew him or her or through public record reviews. Milwaukee's Department of City Development prepared reports listing the racial composition of each aldermanic district using census data. CBO board of directors' racial composition was obtained from the board of directors reports that they were required to submit to CBGA. CBOs were classified as being African American, Caucasian, or other based on the board of directors' racial majority. The racial composition of CBOs' employees was obtained from the Staff Roster reports that CBOs were required to submit to CBGA. Subcontracting data were obtained from the subcontracting reports CBOs were required to submit to CBGA.

References

Abramson, Alan J. and Tobin, Mitchell S. (1994). The changing geography of metropolitan opportunity: The segregation of the poor in the U.S. metropolitan areas, 1970 to 1990. Paper presented at the Fannie Mae Annual Housing Conference. Washington, DC.

Affirmative Action Consulting LTD., Moore, Ralph G., and Associates (1992). *M/WBE disparity study for the County of Milwaukee, City of Milwaukee and Milwaukee Public Schools.* Chicago, IL: Author.

"An era of achievement and neglect" (1988, April 17). *Milwaukee Journal,* p. A1.

"Bank access limited for minorities, report said." (1995, April 10). *Milwaukee Journal,* p. B1.

Beauregard, Robert A. (1990). Tenacious inequalities: Politics and race in Philadelphia. *Urban Affairs Quarterly,* 25(3), 420-434.

Bell, Derrick A. Jr. (1980). *Race, racism, and American law.* Boston, MA: Little, Brown and Company.

Binkley, Lisa S. and White, Sammis B. (1991). *Milwaukee, 1979-1989: A decade of change.* Milwaukee, WI: University of Wisconsin-Milwaukee Urban Research Center.

Blumenfield, Barbara S. (1988). *The Community Development Block Grant program—Milwaukee.* Milwaukee, WI: Legislative Reference Bureau (LRB).

Bobo, Lawrence and Gilliam, Franklin Jr. (1990). Race, sociopolitical participation, and black political empowerment. *American Political Science Review,* 84(2), 377-393.

Browning, Rufus P., Marshall, Dale Rogers, and Tabb, David H. (1984). *Protest is not enough: The struggle of blacks and Hispanics for equality in urban politics.* Berkeley, CA: University of California Press.

Bryner, Gary C. (1987). *Bureaucratic discretion.* New York: Pergamon Press Incorporation.

Bunce, Harold L. and Glickman, Norman J. (1980). The spatial dimensions of the Community Development Block Grant Program: Targeting and urban impacts. In Glickman, Norman J. (Ed.), *The urban impacts of federal policies* (pp. 515-541). Baltimore, MD: John Hopkins University Press.

Bunce, Harold L. and Goldberg, Robert L. (1979). *City need and community development funding.* Washington, DC: United States Department of Housing and Urban Development, Office of Policy Development and Research.

Carmichael, Stokley and Hamilton, Charles V. (1967). *Black power: The politics of liberation in America.* New York: Random House.

Cingranelli, David L. (1981). Race, politics, and elites: Testing alternative models of municipal service distribution. *American Journal of Political Science,* 25(4), 664-692.

"City to use grant to close out WCC properties" (1996, October 5). *Milwaukee Journal Sentinel,* p. B1.

Combs, Michael W. (1995). The Supreme Court, African Americans and public policy: Changes and transformations. In Perry, Huey L. and Parent, Wayne (Eds.), *Blacks and the American political system.* Gainesville, FL: University Press of Florida.

Community Block Grant Administration (CBGA) (1980). *Ollie report.* Milwaukee, WI: Author.

Community Block Grant Administration (CBGA) (1985). *Ollie report.* Milwaukee, WI: Author.

Community Block Grant Administration (CBGA) (1990). *Ollie report.* Milwaukee, WI: Author.

Community Block Grant Administration (CBGA) (1991). *Housing production handbook.* Milwaukee, WI: Author.

Community Block Grant Administration (CBGA) (1993-1997). *CDBG briefing books.* Milwaukee, WI: Author.

Community Block Grant Administration (CBGA) (1995a). *CDBG Milwaukee: Revitalizing the heart of Milwaukee.* Milwaukee, WI: Author .

Community Block Grant Administration (CBGA) (1995b). *Ollie report.* Milwaukee, WI: Author.

Community Block Grant Administration (CBGA) (1996a). *CDBG briefing book.* Milwaukee, WI: Author.

Community Block Grant Administration (CBGA) (1996b). *Housing producers 1995 units completion report.* Milwaukee, WI: Author.

Community Relations-Social Development Commission (CR-SDC) and the Milwaukee Urban League (MUL) (1970). *Black powerlessness in Milwaukee institutions and decision-making structure.* Milwaukee, WI: Milwaukee Urban League.

Comptroller's Office (March, 1996). *Annual review of lending practices of financial institutions.* Milwaukee, WI: Author.

Conta and Associates Inc. (1990). *A study to identify discriminatory practices in the Milwaukee construction marketplace.* Milwaukee, WI: Author.

Cross, Theodore (1987). *The black power imperative: Racial inequality and the politics of nonviolence.* New York: Faulkner Books.

Davidson, Chandler (1984). *Minority vote dilution.* Washington, DC: Howard University Press.

Dedman, Bill. (1989, January 22). Blacks turned down for home loans from s&ls twice as often as Caucasians. *Atlanta Journal-Constitution,* pp. 1, 5.

Derfner, Armand (1984). Vote dilution and the Voting Rights Act amendments of 1982. In Davidson, Chandler (Ed.), *Minority vote dilution* (pp. 145-163). Washington, DC: Howard University Press.

Dommel, Paul R. (1980). Social targeting in community development. *Political Science Quarterly,* 95(3), 465-478.

Dommel, Paul R. (1984). Local discretion: The CDBG approach. In Bingham, Richard D. and Blair, John P. (Eds.), *Urban economic development* (pp. 101-113). Beverly Hills, CA: Sage Publications.

Dommel, Paul R. and Associates (1982). *Decentralizing urban policy: Case studies in community development.* Washington, DC: The Brookings Institution.

Dommel, Paul R. and Rich, Michael J. (1987). The rich get richer: The attenuation of targeting effects of the Community Development Block Grant Program. *Urban Affairs Quarterly,* 22(4), 552-579.

Dries, Mike (1996, July 13). Do nonprofit rehabs need a rehab? *Business Journal,* pp. 1,10.

Edari, Ronald S. (1977). The structure of racial inequality in the Milwaukee area. In Blair, John P. and Edari, Ronald S. (Eds.), *Milwaukee's economy: Market forces, community problems and federal policies* (pp. 86-111). Chicago, IL: The Federal Reserve Bank of Chicago.

Eisinger, Peter K. (1976). *Patterns of interracial politics.* New York: Academic Press, Incorporated.

Eisinger, Peter K. (1982). Black employment in municipal jobs: The impact of black political power. *American Political Science Review,* 76, 380-392.

Eisinger, Peter K. (1991). *City government and minority economic opportunity: The case of Milwaukee.* Madison, WI: University of Wisconsin-Madison, Lafollette Institute of Public Affairs.

Ellison, Charles, Stever, Cynthia, and Stever, James A. (1986). Community Development Block Grants in urban counties: The case of Hamilton County, Ohio. *Journal of Urban Affairs,* 8(1), 72-86.

Enriquez, Darryl (1995, January 30). No general assistance money in sight. *Milwaukee Journal,* p. B1.

Feagin, Joe R., Orum, Anthony M., and Sjoberg, Gideon (Eds.) (1991). *A case for the cases study.* Chapel Hill, NC: University of North Carolina Press.

Frey, William H. (1994). Black college grads, Those in poverty take different migration paths. *Population Today,* 22(2), 1A-2A, 6A.

Garvey, Gerald (1993). *Facing the bureaucracy.* San Francisco, CA: Jossey-Bass Inc.

Gilbert, Craig (1991, March 1). Segregation: Census shows city still surrounded by a white ring. *Milwaukee Journal,* pp. A1, A16.

Gilmer, Jay (1995, January 22). City holds lead in dubious area of loan denials. *Milwaukee Journal,* pp. J1-J2.

Gleiber, Dennis W. and Steger, Mary A. (1983). Decentralization, local priorities, and the Community Development Block Grant Program in Milwaukee. *Publius,* 13(3), 39-55.

Gould, Whitney (1996, June 30). ESHAC to lose houses, sell others: Agency to concentrate on other community housing projects. *Milwaukee Journal Sentinel,* p. B1.

Green, Charles and Wilson, Basil (1989). *The struggle for black empowerment in New York City.* New York: Prater Press.

Gruberg, Martin (1990). Perennial mayor Henry Maier and the Milwaukee political tradition: A case study in urban leadership. Unpublished manuscript, University of Wisconsin-Oshkosh, Oshkosh, Wisconsin.

Gurda, John (1999). *The making of Milwaukee.* Milwaukee, WI: Milwaukee County Historical Society.

Hall, John Stuart (1982). Phoenix, Arizona. In Dommel, Paul R. and Associates (Eds.), *Decentralizing urban policy: Case studies in community development* (pp. 47-83). Washington, DC: The Brookings Institution.

Hall, John Stuart (1983). Fitting the Community Development Block Grant Program to local politics: Who is the tailor? *Publius,* 13(3), 73-84.

Hanks, Lawrence J. (1987). *The struggle for black political empowerment in three Georgia counties.* Knoxville, TN: University of Tennessee Press.

Harrigan, John J. (1989). *Political change in the metropolis,* Fourth edition. Glenview, IL: Scott, Freeman, and Company.

Headley, Bernard D. (1985). Black political empowerment and urban crime. *Pylon,* 46(3), 193-204.

Held, Tom (1995, January 10). Wide racial gap in lending continues. *Milwaukee Sentinel,* p. 5A.

Holt, Mikel (1994, February 23). Milwaukee among most segregated cities in U.S. *Milwaukee Community Journal,* pp. 1, 13.

ICF Incorporated (1992). *Welcome HOME: An introduction to the HOME program.* Fairfax, VA: Author.

"Income gaps widens, report finds" (1995, April 16). *Milwaukee Journal,* p. B1.

Jargowsky, Paul A. (1994). Ghetto poverty among blacks in the 1980s. *Journal of Policy Analysis and Management,* 13(2), 288-310.

Jaynes, Gerald D. and Williams, Robin M. (Eds.) (1989). *A common destiny: Blacks and American society.* Washington, DC: National Academy Press.

Johnson-Elie, Tannette (1996, January 25). Statistics belie efforts at managerial diversity here: Black professionals find better opportunities in other cities. *Milwaukee Journal,* pp. 1, 1D-2D.

Jones, Bryan D. (1981). Party and bureaucracy: The influence of intermediary groups on urban public service delivery. *American Political Science Review,* 75, 668-700.

Jones, Mack H. (1978). Black political empowerment in Atlanta: Myth and reality. *Annals of American Academy of Political and Social Science,* 439, 90-117.

Joshi, Pradnya (1994, October 16). Blacks' road to success leads out of city. *Milwaukee Journal,* pp. 1, 24D-25D.

Judd, Dennis R. and Mushkatel, Alvin H. (1982). Inequality of urban services: The impact of the community development act. In Rich, Richard C. (Ed.), *The politics of urban public services* (pp. 127-139). Washington, DC: Heath and Company.

Kasarda, John D. (1993). Inner-city concentrated poverty and neighborhood distress: 1970 to 1990. Paper Presented at Fannie Mae Annual Housing Conference, Washington, DC.

Knowles, Louis L. and Prewitt, Kenneth (1969). *Institutional racism in America.* Englewood Cliffs, NJ: Prentice-Hall.

Kole, John W. (1987, January 15). Jobless rate high for blacks here, 27.9% figure among worst. *Milwaukee Journal,* pp.1B, 5B.

Legislative Reference Bureau (1994). *Committees and boards book.* Milwaukee, WI: Author.

Levine, Marc V. and Zipp, John F. (1994). *Downtown redevelopment in Milwaukee: Has it delivered for the city?* Milwaukee, WI: University of Wisconsin-Milwaukee Center for Economic Development.

Liebschutz, Sarah F. (1983). Neighborhood conservation: Political choices under the Community Development Block Grant program. *Publius,* 13(3), 23-37.

Lovell, Catherine (1983). Community Development Block Grant: The role of federal requirements. *Publius,* 13(3), 85-97.

MacManus, Susan A. (1990). Minority business contracting with local government. *Urban Affairs Quarterly,* 25(3), 455-473.

Madison, Alvin and Squires, Gregory D. (1996, April 19). African Americans and Latinos robbed by housing industries: Discrimination in the market prevents these two groups from becoming homeowners. *Milwaukee Journal Sentinel,* My Opinion section.

Martin, Michael (1996). Socioeconomic distress in Milwaukee's African American communities, 1980-1990: An analysis of selected demographic variables. Unpublished Master's Thesis, University of Wisconsin-Milwaukee Urban Studies Department, Milwaukee, Wisconsin.

Massey, Douglas S. and Denton, Nancy A. (1989). Hypersegregation in U.S. metropolitan areas: Black and Hispanic segregation along five dimensions. *Demography,* 26(3), 373-391.

Massey, Douglas S. and Denton, Nancy A. (1993). *American apartheid: Segregation and the making of the underclass.* Cambridge, MA: Harvard University Press.

McNeely, R.L. and Kinlow, Melvin R. (1987). *Milwaukee today: A racial gap study.* Milwaukee, WI: Milwaukee Urban League.

Merriam, Sharan B. (1990). *Case study research in education: A qualitative approach.* San Francisco: Jossey-Bass Inc.

Mitchell, Thomas E. (1994, March 2). City providing example, aide to mayor declares. *Milwaukee Community Journal,* pp. 1, 9.

Morris, Milton D. (1984). Black electoral participation and the distribution of public benefits. In Davidson, Chandler (Ed), *Minority vote dilution* (pp. 271-285). Washington, DC: Howard University Press.

Murphy, Mary Beth (1994a, February 28). Jobs key for blacks on move: Few professionals choose Milwaukee. *Milwaukee Sentinel,* p. 4A.

Murphy, Mary Beth (1994b, February 28). Milwaukee prime place for poor blacks who move. *Milwaukee Sentinel,* pp. 1A, 4A.

Nathan, Richard P., Dommel, Paul R., Liebschutz, Sarah F., Morris, Milton D., and Associates (1977). *Block grants for community development.* Washington, DC: United States Department of Housing and Urban Development (HUD).

Nichols, Mike (1993a, September 26). Blacks' jobless rate is 2nd highest in U.S. *Milwaukee Journal,* pp. 1B, 7B.

Nichols, Mike (1993b, September 24). Joblessness still plagues blacks in city. *Milwaukee Journal,* pp. 1, 10.

Nichols, Mike (1995a, March 26). Disparity in home values further divides city: For many central city residents, it means less equity. *Milwaukee Journal,* pp. 1A-2A.

Nichols, Mike (1995b, January 18). Neighbors want housing group evicted. *Milwaukee Journal,* p. B1.

Nichols, Mike (1998, May 23). City gives ESHAC last opportunity. *Milwaukee Journal Sentinel,* p. B1.

Norman, Jack (1993, October 3). Central city lending up, but race gap widens. *Milwaukee Journal,* pp. 1D-2D.

Norman, Jack (1995, October 6). Emotions high at hearings on use of federal grants. City has $36.6 million to ease such needs as emergency housing. *Milwaukee Journal Sentinel,* p. B3.

Norman, Jack (1996a, September 17). Housing agency's troubles expensive hundreds of thousand dollars misspent, Gordon says. *Milwaukee Journal Sentinel,* p. A1.

Norman, Jack (1996b, January 21). Inner city still trails in lending. *Milwaukee Journal Sentinel,* pp. 1B, 3B.

Norman, Jack (1996c, November 9). Norquist vetoes block grant money for SDC. *Milwaukee Journal Sentinel,* pp. B1, B4.

Norman, Jack (1996d, February 29). Talks break down ESHAC faces loss of homes. Foreclosure expected on 28 houses owned by community group. *Milwaukee Journal Sentinel,* p. A1.

Norman, Jack (1997a, February 22). City puts housing contracts with ESHAC on hold. *Milwaukee Journal Sentinel,* pp. B1, B4.

Norman, Jack (1997b, March 6). ESHAC's repayment plans are rejected: Comptroller tells agency to return $66,000 now. *Milwaukee Journal Sentinel,* p. B1.

Norman, Jack (1997c, March 8). Housing agency gets lease on life. *Milwaukee Journal Sentinel,* p. B1.

Norman, Jack (1997d, March 1). Progress seen in housing snarl. *Milwaukee Journal Sentinel,* p. B1.

Norman, Jack (1997e, February 23). Renter's nightmare: Sewage backup sickens child as agencies remained mired in dispute. *Milwaukee Journal Sentinel,* pp. B1, B12.

Norman, Jack and Borowski, Greg J. (1999, March 21). Where have all the houses gone? *Milwaukee Journal Sentinel,* pp. A1, A5.

Norman, Jack and Daykin, Tom (1996, January 27). Missing payments, ESHAC sued by local lenders settlement may be reached next week. *Milwaukee Journal Sentinel,* p. B1.

O'Hare, William (1986). The best metros for blacks. *American Demographics,* 8, 27-33.

Orlebeke, Charles J. (1983). CDBG in Chicago: The politics of control. *Publius,* 13(3), 57-72.

Parker, Frank R. (1990). *Black votes count: Political empowerment in Mississippi after 1965.* Chapel Hill, NC: University of North Carolina Press.

Patton, Michael Quinn (1990). *Qualitative evaluation and research methods,* Second edition. Newbury Park, CA: Sage Publications.

Perry, Huey L. (1980). The socioeconomic impact of black political empowerment in a rural southern locality. *Rural Sociology,* 45(2), 207-222.

Perry, Huey L. and Parent, Wayne (Eds.) (1995). *Blacks and the American political system.* Gainesville, FL: University Press of Florida.

Peterson, Paul E., Rabe, Barry G., and Wong, Kenneth K. (1986). *When federalism works.* Washington, DC: The Brookings Institution.

Piliawsky, Monte (1985, Spring). The impact of black mayors on the black community: The case of New Orleans' Ernest Morial. *Review of Black Political Economy,* 13(4), 5-23.

Piven, Frances F. and Clowards, Richard A. (1971). Black control of cities. In Greenberg, Edward, Milner, Neal, and Olson, David J. (Eds.), *Black politics, the inevitability of conflict: Readings* (pp. 118-130). New York: Holt, Rinehart, and Winston.

Pohlmann, Marcus D. (1990). *Black politics in conservative America.* New York: Longman Press.

Proceedings of the Common Council (1975-1976, 1988-1989, and 1991-1992). Milwaukee, WI: City Clerk's Office.

Rich, Michael J. (1993). *Federal policymaking and the poor.* Princeton, NJ: Princeton University Press.

Robinson, Carla Jean (1990). Minority political representation and local economic development policy. *Journal of Urban Affairs,* 12(1), 49-57.

Rose, Harold M. (1992). *The employment status of young black males residing in poverty households: Recent Milwaukee County experience.* Milwaukee, WI: University of Wisconsin-Milwaukee Employment and Training Institute.

Rose, Harold M., Edari, Ronald S., Quinn, Lois M., and Pawasarat, John (1992). *The labor market experience of young African American men from low-income families in Wisconsin.* Milwaukee, WI: University of Wisconsin-Milwaukee Employment and Training Institute.

Rosenfeld, Raymond A. (1980). Who benefits and who decides? The uses of Community Development Block Grants. In Rosenthal, Donald B. (Ed.), *Urban revitalization* (pp. 211-235). Beverly Hills, CA: Sage Publications.

Ross, Bernell L. (1994, June 11). Agency's full disclosures are not fully disclosed. *Milwaukee Courier Newspaper,* pp. 1, 19.

Rummler, Gary C. (1986, June 19). Financially city Blacks rank poorly. *Milwaukee Journal,* p. 1B.

Sacco, John F. (1982). Community distribution of federal funds: The Community Development Block Grant Program. In Rich, Richard C. (Ed.), *The politics of urban public services* (pp. 141-156). Washington, DC: Heath and Company.

Schmandt, Henry J., Wendel, George D., and Otte, George (1983). CDBG continuity or change? *Publius,* 13(3), 7-23.

Schuldt, Gretchen (1997a, February 24). Home rehab group had runaway costs. *Milwaukee Journal Sentinel,* pp. B1, B7.

Schuldt, Gretchen (1997b, February 21). Rehab agency cost city $1.4 million. *Milwaukee Journal Sentinel,* pp. A1, A8.

Schuldt, Gretchen (1997c, March 3). Westside Conservation leaves legacy both bad and good. *Milwaukee Journal Sentinel,* pp. B1, B7.

Schuldt, Gretchen (1997d, March 2). Westside Conservation work focus on duplex owner's claim. *Milwaukee Journal Sentinel,* pp. B1, B7.

Squires, Gregory D. (1993, December 16-23). Response to shrinking the racial gap: "Wait." *Shepherd Express,* p. 3.

Squires, Gregory D. (1994). *Capital and communities in black and white: The intersections of race, class, and uneven development.* Albany, NY: State University of New York-Albany Press.

Squires, Gregory D. and O'Connor, Sally (1998). Fringe banking in Milwaukee: The rise of check cashing businesses and the emergence of a two-tiered banking system. *Urban Affairs Review,* 34(1), 126-149.

Squires, Gregory D. and Velez, William (1987). Insurance redlining and the transformation of an urban metropolis. *Urban Affairs Quarterly,* 23(1), 63-83.

Steger, Mary Ann (1984). Group influence versus decision-making rules: An analysis of local CDBG allocational decisions. *Urban Affairs Quarterly,* 19(3), 373-394.

Thomas, Clayton John (1986). The personal side of street-level bureaucracy: Discrimination or neutral competence? *Urban Affairs Quarterly,* 22(1), 84-100.

Tuerina, Edmund S. (1993, March 11). Racial division: City is still a case study in segregation: Report gives Milwaukee dubious distinction as "hypersegregated." *Milwaukee Journal,* p. B1.

Umhoefer, David E. (1988, April 6). Victors' vision of unity: Norquist to open doors to minorities. *Milwaukee Journal,* p. B1.

U.S. Department of Commerce, Bureau of Census, Census of Population and Housing, Milwaukee, Wisconsin (1970, 1975 Special Census, 1980 and 1990). Washington, DC: Author.

U.S. Department of Housing and Urban Development (HUD) (1996). *Everything you ever needed to know about the CDBG Program.* Washington, DC: Author.

Walters, Steven. (1988, May 2). Norquist shaking up boards. *Milwaukee Sentinel,* p. A1.

White, Jack E. (1992, May 11). The limits of black power. *Time,* pp. 38-40.

Williams, Linda F. (1990). White/black perceptions of the electability of black candidates. In Barker, Lucius, J. (Ed.), *Black electoral politics* (pp. 45-64). New Brunswick, NJ: Transaction Publisher.

Wilson, William Julius (1996). *When work disappears.* New York: Alfred A. Knopf.

Wisconsin Council on Children and Families. (1994, July). The growing concentration of African American poverty in Milwaukee, pp. 1-4.

Wong, Kenneth K. and Peterson, Paul E. (1986). Urban response to federal program flexibility: Politics of Community Development Block Grant. *Urban Affairs Quarterly,* 21(3), 293-309.

Yin, Robert K. (1994). *Case study research: Design and methods,* Second edition. Thousand Oaks, CA: Sage Publications.

Yinger, John. (1995). *Closed doors, opportunities lost: The continuing costs of housing discrimination.* New York: Russell Sage Foundation.

Index

Abramson, Alan J., 30
ACT Landmark Housing, 95, 96
African Americans
    bias against, in CDBG funding
        process, 75-78
    as elected officials, 7-8
    increased presence in political
        machinery of government, 3-5
    political power
        in Atlanta, Georgia, 7
        effect on municipal resources, 1
        factors limiting, 6-7
    socioeconomic status in Milwaukee
        city residence, 29
        elimination of General
            Assistance Program, 31
        high concentration in low-paying
            jobs, 37
        home values, 35-36
        loan rejection rates, 34-35
        low concentration in professional
            jobs, 36-37
        minority-owned businesses,
            37-38
        population growth, 29
        poverty rates, 29-31
        revitalization projects, 36
        segregation, 32-33
        unemployment rates, 31-32
    voter registration, 4-6
Agape, 95
Aid for Families with Dependent
    Children (AFDC), 30-31
Atlanta, Georgia, political structure, 7

Baltimore, Maryland, 17
Beauregard, Robert A., 6

Bilandic, Michael, 17
Brown v. Board of Education, 3-4
Bunce, Harold L., 20
Byrne, Jane, 17

Carpenter's Incorporated, 77, 94-95
CBGA *Briefing Book,* 81, 83, 84
CBOs. *See* community-based
    organizations (CBOs)
CD float, 16
CDBG. *See* community development
    block grant (CDBG)
CDBG *Briefing Book,* 79, 80, 84
Chicago, Illinois, 17, 21
CHPC. *See* Community Housing and
    Preservation Corporation
    (CHPC)
citizen advisory committee (CAC), 22
Civil Rights Act of 1957, 4
Civil Rights Act of 1964, 4
civil servants, role in distribution of
    CDBG funds, 19-20
color line, 1
Commandos Incorporation, 79-80, 107
common council
    role in distribution of CDBG funds,
        18
    strength of mayor via, 18-19
community block grant administration
    (CBGA), 25-26
community development block grant
    (CDBG)
    defined, 1
    overview, 13-27
        CBOs and, 20-21
        citizen participation, 22-23
        civil servants' influence, 19-20

community development block grant
(CDBG), overview
(continued)
common councils' roles in
distribution of funds, 18
consolidation of previous
programs, 13-14
hands-off versus hands-on
approaches, 14-15
leveraging devices, 15-16
mayors' roles in distribution of
funds, 16-18
national objectives, 14
need indicators, 20
research, 22-25
as reform and consolidation
measure, 1-2
Community Development Policy
Committee (CDPC), 2, 25-26
Community Housing and Preservation
Corp (CHPC), 85
Community Organizing Westside
Agency (COWSA), 91
community-based organizations
(CBOs), 2, 3
negative influence of race in
allocation of CDBG funds,
43-51
preferential treatment of African
Americans in allocation of
CDBG funds, 40-43
role in distribution of CDBG funds,
20-21

Daley, Richard, 17
Daley, Richard Jr., 17
Denton, Nancy A., 32
Donegan, Tom, 10
DuBois, W. E. B., 1

East Side Housing Action Committee
(ESHAC), 82, 85-88, 107, 111
Edari, Ronald S., 37
Eisenhower, Dwight, 4

Equal Employment Opportunity
Commission (EEOC), 36
ESHAC. *See* East Side Housing Action
Committee (ESHAC)

Faubus, Orville, 4
Fighting Back Initiative, 98-99
finance and personnel committee
(F&P), 26
funding allocation plan (FAP), 26

Goldberg, Robert L., 20
Guinn v. United States, 3

Henningsen, Paul, 10
Home Ownership Made Easy (HOME),
83
HOME Program, 96-97, 98, 111
Housing Partnership Corporation
(HPC), 86
HUD. *See* United States Department of
Housing and Urban
Development

Inner City Redevelopment Corporation
(ICRC), 47

Jackson, Maynard, 7
Jim Crow system, 1, 3
Jones, Bryan D., 19
Journey House, 95-96

Levine, Marc V., 37

MacManus, Susan A., 6
Maier, Henry, 9, 10, 24, 50, 55-65,
101-2, 104
Martin, Michael, 32

Martin Luther King (MLK)
Incorporation, 99
Massey, Douglas S., 32
mayors
roles in distribution of CDBG funds,
16-18
strength of, via common council,
18-19
techniques used to dominate CDBG
program, 16
McNamara-McGraw, Lorraine, 10
McNulty, Mary Anne, 10
Milwaukee, Wisconsin
bending existing CDBG rules, 91-99
carryover funds, 91-93
HOME program, 96-97, 98
reprogramming dollars, 93-96
CDBG allocation patterns, 55-74
aldermanic districts, 56-65
economic development projects,
71-72
housing projects, 65-71
during Maier's administration,
55-65
during Norquist's administration,
63-74
proposal recommendations,
55-56
public service projects, 72-73
citizen participation plan, 22
Council Resolution number 74-92,
25
demographic and political changes,
8-11
distribution of CDBG funds, 2
funding allocation plan, 26
research studies, 23-25
triage approach, 23
impact of race in allocation of
CDBG funds, 39-54, 75-89
benefits and drawbacks of CDBG
program, 51-54
bias against African Americans,
75-78
CDBG-funded city jobs, 49

Milwaukee, Wisconsin, impact of race
in allocation of CDBG funds
(continued)
direct effects, 101-12
practice of terminating cash
advances, 78-89
preferential treatment
perspective, 40-43
race as negative influence
perspective, 43-51
survey respondents' opinions,
39-40
socioeconomic status of African
Americans, 29-38
city residence, 29
elimination of General
Assistance Program, 31
high concentration in low-paying
jobs, 37
home values, 35-36
loan rejection rates, 34-35
low concentration in professional
jobs, 36-37
minority-owned businesses,
37-38
population growth, 29
poverty rates, 29-31
revitalization projects, 36
segregation, 32-33
unemployment rates, 31-32
Milwaukee Christian Center, 95
Milwaukee Housing Assistance
Corporation (MHAC), 48
Milwaukee United for Better Housing
(MUFBH), 66, 80-81, 92
municipal resources, effect of African-
American political power on, 1

need indicators, 20
neighborhood advisory council (NAC),
22
New Covenant, 93, 107
Nonprofit Center, 96

Norquist, John O., 9-10, 55, 63-74, 101-2, 104-5, 106
North Division Resident Association, 44-46
Northwest Side Community Development Corporation (NWSCDC), 47-48, 82, 88-89, 106, 107, 111

O. C. White Soul Club, 46, 81-82, 107

Pawasarat, John, 37
Project Respect, 46-47

Quinn, Lois M., 37

Redevelopment Authority of the City of Milwaukee (RACM), 85
Rochester, New York, 21
Rose, Harold M., 37

Schaefer, William Donald, 17
Schreiber, Martin, 9
Smith v. Allwright, 3
Social Development Commission (SDC), 75-77
South Carolina v. Katzenbach, 4
Southside Community Organization (SCO), 91
Squires, Gregory D., 33
Steger, Mary Ann, 23-24

targeted investment neighborhood (TIN), 95-96
Tobin, Mitchell S., 30

United States Department of Housing and Urban Development (HUD), 1, 18, 20
citizen participation stipulation, 22
funding caps, 26
review and monitoring, 21

Velez, William, 33
Voting Rights Act of 1965, 4-5

Washington, Harold, 17
Westside Conservation Corporation (WCC), 48, 82-85, 106, 107, 111
Wisconsin Council on Children and Families, 30

Yinger, John, 33
Young, Andrew, 7

Zipp, John F., 37
zoning, neighborhoods, and development committee (ZN&D), 26, 98